The Cure Within

Lubomir Bic

Zuzana Bic

ISBN-10: 1986389219
ISBN-13: 978-1986389211

I died twenty-three years ago. Not clinically, but more like a plant that has been ripped out of the ground. While its leaves are still green and firm, betraying none of the events that will soon follow, this is a plant condemned to a certain death. In a few hours, its crown will begin to sag; its leaves will curl up and turn brown. It will cease to exist. It is not its immediate appearance that pronounced the death sentence but the finality of time remaining.

I died twenty-three years ago. It was an unusually hot day in late March, a Monday. I remember it vividly, in the way we remember all momentous events in life. The death sentence was handed down to me by Dr. Green, California's premier oncologist at the UCMA Medical Center.

"I am afraid I have some bad news today," he said, raising his tired eyes from a medical file spread in front of him. He was calm, his voice professionally reassuring.

"The cancer is in its very advanced stage," he elaborated cautiously, "it has metastasized and invaded several vital organs."

Dr. Green continued his monologue for a while, laying out my various options.

"Six to eight months," he confirmed glumly when I asked about my future.

Six to eight months to live. I was desperately trying to concentrate on his speech but my mind kept tearing itself away in frantic bursts of panic. I was capturing frightening fragments of medical terminology ... radical chemotherapy ... radiation ... life expectancy. Life expectancy! There was no hope of recovery, only a desperate fight to steal a few more months on this earth, tied to a hospital, then to a hospital bed, then ...

As I left the air-conditioned building and walked into the hot air, my body broke into a clammy sweat. I walked to my car in a state of befuddled daze, punctuated by spasms of oppressing anguish. I let myself drop into the leather upholstery, turned the air conditioning to max, and leaned my head back into the headrest. As I sat there, numb and exhausted, I understood what someone facing eminent death always says: my entire life passed in front of my closed eyes as a silent movie.

Until a few moments ago, I took my existence for granted. I considered myself successful and reasonably happy. Now, nothing made sense. Success—what an illusion. I would trade everything for a reversal of my misfortune. I would gladly become a beggar, an outcast, a criminal, even a slave, if only I could erase Dr. Green's death sentence.

I must have sat there for an hour, absentmindedly watching people enter and leave the building. I only had six months to live and no idea what to do during that time. Mechanically, I put the car in gear and drove home in a daze. There I lay on the sofa in the living room and stared at the white ceiling.

I wondered why people have such an insatiable desire to see into the future. Is it so that they could change the events that lie ahead? During the eons before science they resorted to witchcraft, sorcery, or soothsaying to presage what lay ahead. Today, we deploy the latest diagnostic technology. Yet, paradoxically, it is the unknown that keeps us alive.

For a child, life is endless. As we mature, we begin to grasp our mortality. We know that someday all must part, but that someday is undefined. We could die today or live until the age of one-hundred. And even then, life is still open-ended. As long as we don't know the moment of death, we are alive.

I must have fallen asleep. When I opened my eyes, it was already nighttime. I was still on the sofa, fully dressed, and lacking the willpower to get up. I began to sweat again. It was a cold, unpleasant sweat that made me shiver. I crossed my arms on my chest and stared into the darkness. I was facing the biggest fear of my life and I was alone. No one could do or say anything to make me feel better. I could see the end of my journey.

I knew that I should get up, take a shower, go to bed. But did it matter? Nothing really mattered anymore.

I fell asleep again but woke up a few hours later in the same state of desperation and total hopelessness. Why bother getting up, going to work, or doing anything at all?

At 10 am I finally dragged myself up, went to the bathroom, and washed my face. I looked into the mirror and saw a face worn down to a waxy mask of sorrow. I filled a bowl with cornflakes, poured over some milk, and began to eat it mechanically while staring out the window. I asked myself if I should still prune the peach tree in the garden as I did every year?

I decided to analyze my options rationally. There were only two. I could try to extend my life by every precious minute that the doctors, through the marvels of modern medicine, would help me steal from Dr. Death. That meant spending the rest of my days tied to a hospital and hoping to still be alive the next day. Or I could try to squeeze out every ounce of meaning from the days I still had left. But what would I like to do? I had money, but not enough to leave behind a serious legacy of charitable acts. I had no close family to deal with, no loose ends to tie up. The idea of a "bucket list" came to my mind— why not just do whatever I felt doing for as long as I could— do a parachute jump, climb the Kilimanjaro, dive with the sharks on the Great Barrier Reef, buy a Ferrari, eat meals I never wanted to waste money on, or maybe try some drugs…

In the end, I passed the day by doing nothing. The night was endless as I kept floating between states of unrewarding semi-sleep and numbing wakefulness. Why would anyone like to know the future?

***

I was still lying on the sofa, staring into empty space and ceaselessly rolling over the same boulders of dark thoughts in a Sisyphean nightmare when the phone rang. It startled me, then it upset me. Doesn't everyone know? I don't want to talk to any compassionate relative or friend; and most definitely not to some telemarketer. But wait—maybe it's the hospital; there has been some grave mistake, the wrong diagnosis. My heart was pounding when I reluctantly picked up the receiver. A friendly male voice asked to speak with me but the mispronunciation of my name just added to my irritation. I hung up. I didn't need life insurance or whatever he was selling.

The phone rang again a minute later. I let it ring but the caller was persistent.

"Yes?" I said angrily as I picked up again.

The same voice asks for me, this time pronouncing my name correctly.

"This is he," I acknowledged.

"I am very sorry to intrude but I need to speak with you." He spoke politely but with an unmistakable tone of urgency.

"What about?"

"I would like to talk to you about … your condition."

I became alert.

"Are you from the clinic," I asked.

"Oh no, not from the clinic." He hesitated for an instant. "But I happen to know."

"How—" I tried to interrupt but he continued unperturbed.

"Please do not ask me how, or why, not now. That's not so important. The only thing that matters is that you do not have much time. You need to act." He waited for my reply.

"Who the hell are you?" I asked. "You are not from the clinic, you know something you shouldn't know—there are laws, you know. You call out of the blue—how did you get my number anyway?"

"I'm sorry."

"You are sorry? About what? Disturbing me? You don't even tell me who you are but urge me to act when the doctors have given up?"

I was beginning to think that this was some other telemarketing efforts, perhaps trying to sell me a cemetery plot or a discount on cremation. Sick bastards. I was about to hang up again when his voice came back.

"Please don't hang up on me. Just hear me out. What do you have to lose?"

There was a profound truth in his question. What does one

have to lose after death?

"Ok. What do you want?" I asked, still on edge.

"I only want to help you," he said.

I rolled my eyes. "Please, get to the point. What are you selling?"

"Life," he said.

"Life? Not life insurance? I thought only God can grant life. Are you God?"

"Only God can grant life," he replied, "but you already have yours. You do not need another one. What you need is to hold on to the one you have."

This guy was not an ordinary salesman. His answers did not follow any protocol. He was a philosopher.

"And you can help me hold on to my life?" I asked.

"Most likely." He said this with such confidence that I sat up to better concentrate.

"Are you a doctor, or a healer, or a shaman, or...? "

"I am a former patient." He remained silent for a few seconds to let the words sink in. "I too had cancer. I too was told that my days were numbered and the count was frighteningly low. I too received an anonymous phone call, and I too almost hung up."

After a few more seconds of silence he added, "But that was twenty-three years ago."

"So this is a reference call?" I asked.

"If you wish to call it that. Part of my own cure—in fact the last step of it—was to come back and to help someone else in a similar situation. So that's what I am doing. I am calling you and offering help. If you accept, I will have completed my cure."

How strange, I thought. Could there really be some magic cure somewhere, unknown to or perhaps rejected by the medical establishment? Some secret society of healers, anxiously guarding their secret and only passing it from patient to patient by word of mouth? It sounded just too incredible, too much like a plot for a sinister novel or a film noir. But as I was about to dismiss it all, the harsh reality hit me again: if I do nothing, the doctor's prognosis will surely come true. So no matter what I do, no matter how stupid, naïve, or dangerous my actions, the final outcome could not turn out worse than if I did nothing.

For a long time, my thoughts kept spinning in a hurricane of pros and cons, challenges and regrets, accusations and self-pity. As they began to settle, my anger, frustration, and feelings of powerlessness began to transform themselves into a force urging me to do something, anything, just not give up.

"So what exactly would I have to do?" I asked after a moment of tense silence. "What exactly is this 'cure' you are talking about?"

"I am very happy for you," the voice at the other end said, sounding relieved. "I cannot tell you what the cure is because not knowing is part of it."

That was a bit mysterious for my taste.

"Fine, but what happens next? What should I do?"

"Do you have a backpack? Something not too large," he asked.

"Sure, but—"

He cut me off.

"Please do not ask any more questions. Trust me. Pack some spare clothes and a few daily necessities—toothbrush, comb, a bottle of water, you know, the usual for a casual trip. And take your passport. Then check your mailbox tomorrow morning. That's it. That's all you need to know, ok?"

"Hey, listen—"

"Please don't ask any more. It will all become clear, soon. Trust me, and more importantly, trust yourself. I hope to see you in a few years but now I must leave you. Good luck."

The line went silent. The porthole to the other world was closed.

***

The next morning, my mailbox contained a plain white envelope containing an airline ticket issued in my name. The destination was Addis Ababa, Ethiopia, departing at 9:20 pm, that very same evening. No letter, no further instructions, not even a contact phone number. Defying all rational thought, I grabbed the already packed backpack, took a cab to the airport, and checked in.

The next several hours passed as if in a daze. After getting through the immigration and customs formalities, I walked out into the arrival hall and was met by a young smiling woman who mercifully rescued me from the assault of porters, taxi drivers, and hotel agents who immediately descended upon me as a pack of vultures sensing a weakened prey. Without providing any explanation, she motioned me to follow her. She guided me to another boarding gate where, with another charming smile, she handed me a new boarding pass. Before I realized what was happening, she had already dissolved in the colorful crowd filling every inch of the airport.

I checked the boarding pass. It read: Golunga, departure: 10:05. That was in twenty minutes and a chaotic process of boarding was already under way. I worked my way into the small crowd of passengers and eventually ended up in the window seat of a small turboprop aircraft.

Three hours later, the pilot announced our impending descent into what, from this altitude, appeared to be a quilt of green and brown patches of velvet. A few minutes later, the plane came to a halt on a bumpy narrow landing strip and impatiently taxied to a small arrival hall—the only building constituting the airport's infrastructure.

I passed quickly through the dinky narrow building and began to study the mix of dilapidated taxis, motorcycles, tricycles, rickshaws, and other even more dubious modes of transportation, all of which were clogging the only road in front of the airport. They were all engaged in various stages of greeting, loading, and spiritedly negotiating with the arriving passengers. Not knowing what to do next, I resigned myself to fate, which soon manifested itself in the form of a young man, who suddenly appeared at my side.

"I am Ngome," he said, stretching out his hand to greet me. "Welcome to Golunga,"

"Hi," I replied, trying to appear relaxed.

"I will be your driver."

I was tempted to ask what our next destination might be, but the young man had already picked up my backpack and pointed to what looked like a Jeep or a Land Rover at the end of the line. "Please follow me."

"Where are we going?" I managed to yell as we pushed our way through the unruly crowd toward the SUV.

"I am to take you to your new home," he said.

"My new home?"

"Yes, sir. It's not too far, just a few hours down this road," he elaborated, waving his hand in a noncommittal direction.

"But I am supposed to meet … well … I don't really know. Is there a hospital around here?"

His forehead crinkled in puzzlement. "A hospital, sir?"

"Yes, a hospital or a clinic, or something like that."

He shook his head. "The nearest hospital is in Mwangoro. But that's very far, sir. Over there." He again flicked his wrist toward an elusive point on the horizon.

I sighed and raised myself into the passenger seat of what turned out to be a Land Rover from some much earlier and more glorious past of this country. Ngome turned the key, the powerful V-8 revved up a few times, and we took off in a cloud of brown dust.

A few miles beyond the airport the road began to shed its pavement. It gradually began to assume the appearance of a corrugated roof, which my driver attempted to subdue by speeding up to skim over its crests. I wanted to ask him how long we still had to go, but given the machine-gun-like rattle produced by the gravel hitting the vehicle's underside, any attempt at conversation was futile.

I closed my eyes holding on to the overhead bar with one hand and with the other pushing against the bottom of my seat to maintain balance. Occasionally I glanced at the speedometer. It vibrated heavily around 40, which I assumed were miles per hour.

must have slipped into a state of hypnotic semi-consciousness for it took me by surprise when the car pulled over and slid to a halt in a cloud of dust. At first I thought that something had happened, a mechanical problem or a collision with a wildebeest, but the driver was smiling at me encouragingly.

"We are here, sir," he announced.

I looked around, shielding my eyes against the early afternoon sun. We were surrounded by a landscape of gently rolling hills in shades of copper and gold, dotted by occasional sycamores and baobab trees. I looked at the driver to see if he was trying to joke.

"What do you mean?" I said. "We are in the middle of nowhere."

The driver jumped down and walked around the back of the car to my side. With his arm outstretched, he pointed to a path, not more than two feet wide, that took off from the main road toward the distant mountains.

"You follow this path, sir," he said gingerly. "It will take you straight to your place. You can't miss it."

"But ... how far do I walk? What should I look for?"

He threw up his hands up in the universal gesture of non-commitment.

"I am sorry sir, but those were all my instructions. You are to follow this path."

He fished out a canteen from the trunk of his SUV and slipped its strap over my head, letting it rest against my chest. It was heavy. I felt panicky; I felt an urge to grab his arm and make him take me back. Instead, I froze and just watched as he jumped back into the SUV and spun it around in an avalanche of gravel. He took off in a reddish cloud of dust, waving his outstretched arm in a long goodbye.

I stood there by the road, watching the dust cloud slowly disappear toward the horizon. I shook my head, unable to comprehend what had just happened. I was dying, in desperate need of medical care, yet I stood alone in the middle of some African bush with a small backpack and a canteen of lukewarm drinking water around my neck. If I wanted to die quickly, I could have done that in the comfort of my home. And now the image of my beautiful home overlooking the Pacific Ocean came back to me like a nostalgic flashback from a different life.

I hoisted the backpack over my shoulder and started to walk along the path pointed out by the driver. The sun was still high above my head, making my shadow disappear below my feet. I walked for what felt like a very long time but in reality amounted to barely an hour. I was seriously out of shape and walking as a mode of transportation was totally foreign to me. Back home, the only walks I took were between the elevator near my office and the closest parking spot reserved for the company's privileged few.

I looked around. There had been no noticeable change in the landscape since I started my walk. I was moving through an endless sea of tall golden grass swaying back and forth with each gust of the wind. It was calming, almost hypnotizing, but my mind refused to give in. What if all of this was just some sick joke? What if I keep walking all day and found nothing but the same grass? I stopped to look back. Should I turn around? We must have driven for several hours on that miserable gravel road and didn't pass a single car in either direction. Walking back would be suicide. Walking forward offered some hope.

My thoughts of self-pity were suddenly interrupted by a deep growl. I stopped and, holding my breath, cautiously scanned my surroundings. I became aware of my own heart trying to break out of my chest. Then I spotted her. Just a few yards to my right, partly hidden by the tall grass, stood a lioness. She observed me motionlessly. Her mouth was stained with the blood of her kill in front of her, which she was in the process of devouring. As I stood there looking into her eyes and hypnotized by her stare, I perceived the complete silence surrounding us, disturbed by only the frantic beating of my own heart. I did not know what to do. I remembered someone telling me over a beer in some pub a long time ago that the only dangerous lion was the one you didn't see. Still, I was afraid to move. The lioness resolved the situation by resuming her meal, evidently unimpressed by my presence.

I took a slow tentative step sideways. She displayed no intentions to leave her prey. I made a few more cautious steps at an angle that would gradually increase the distance between us but without appearing to flee. Encouraged by her indifference, I resumed my walk along the path, slow at first, but increasing my pace with each step until I was running as fast as my pathetically unfit body would permit me, and then even a few minutes longer. When I finally came to rest, I had to lean on the trunk of an uprooted tree to steady myself, panting, coughing, and clutching my side to suppress the stabbing pain.

When the panic subsided, I resumed my walk but something had changed in me. I felt strangely animated but could not explain why. Until a moment ago I only had one enemy—my disease. Now there were others vying for my life. I began to wonder which of them would get me first.

I took another sip of water from my bottle, which by now was almost empty. That raised another nagging concern. I kept walking, taking short breaks every hour to rest my feet, which were beginning to show serious signs of chafing. At least I had the foresight to put on tennis shoes this morning.

Toward the late afternoon, the landscape began to gradually change. The path had an ascending tendency, and as I was reaching higher ground, the tones of brown, yellow, and ocher, became displaced by various shades of green. The number and variety of trees and bushes also increased considerably, making it more difficult to see far ahead. My mood took a turn for the better when I came upon a narrow brook, meandering slowly along the path I was following. I knelt down and splashed my face with the refreshingly cool water. I was achingly thirsty but I hesitated for a moment. In my entire life I never drank anything that did not come out of a bottle or a can. I felt like a child breaking an unwritten rule. Do you dare? I sank my head down until my lips touched the surface of the water, and began to drink in long satisfying drafts, feeling the cooling liquid slowly penetrating every cell of my body.

Having quenched my thirst, I rolled over on my back, spreading my arms and legs away from my body and just stared into the milky blue sky above me. I felt tired, aching in places I didn't know could ache, but it felt strangely pleasant and satisfying at the same time. All the worries, commitments, anxieties of the fifty plus years of my existence have receded into the background. Nothing really mattered now. I felt free. Free as all the other living beings I was sharing this moment with, concerned with only the present moment, unwilling to carry the burden of knowing the future.

I closed my eyes, feeling the muscles of my body gradually relaxing and my mind letting go of the thoughts that had paralyzed me during the past two days, until I drifted away into a peaceful sleep. I awoke briefly several times during that night. Each time it took me a moment to realize where I was but, for some reason, the thought of sleeping alone in the middle of Africa did not frighten me any longer. Each time I awoke I just turned over to find a more comfortable position in the soft grass and let the sound of the brook soothe me back to sleep.

I woke up uncomfortably wet. It was still dark and it was raining. Not heavily, but enough to soak my clothes to the skin. I was shivering. I hugged my knees to my chest, trying to keep warm, but it was no use. My teeth were chattering and I had no shelter. I was sure I would catch pneumonia and die much before my cancer had a chance to kill me.

A strange rustle in the grass made me alert. I held my breath to hear better. There were steps in the darkness; slow, shuffling steps, coming closer. Then I saw him—a tall figure silhouetted against the gray sheet of mist descending from the sky. I could not make out his face. He stood a few feet away, dressed in a loose white robe. He was leaning on a spear whose tip stood up to his shoulder. My heart was racing. Should I get up, say something, run?

"Hello my friend," he said in a quiet voice.

I wanted to reply but my throat was choked off by an invisible noose.

"You are shivering," he said. "Why not take off your wet clothes? You will feel much better."

I opened my mouth but no sound came out.

He seemed to smile in the darkness. Then, without saying another word, he turned and slowly walked away.

TI woke up and it took me a moment to realize that I had just dreamt my encounter with the strange man. It was raining—that was no dream—and I was wet down to my underwear, but there was no mysterious visitor. Why did he tell me to take off my clothes?

I rose and wrestled the wet shirt off my body. I wrung it out and threw it over a nearby bush. Then I took off my pants. My boxer shorts were completely wet as well. I hesitated. It felt strange to get naked in the wilderness but I slipped them off too. There were several large trees around me. I walked to the nearest one and felt the ground around its trunk with my feet. It was dry. I lay down close to the base, curled up into a fetal position, raked a few handfuls of dry leaves around my body, and closed my eyes. As my skin began to dry off, my limbs stopped shivering. A few minutes later I was slipping back into sleep.

A cacophony of bird cries and insect chirps woke me up at sunrise. I brushed off the dry leaves that were clinging to my naked body and put on the already dry clothes. I refilled the canteen from the brook and resumed my walk. It didn't take long for me to realize how hungry I was. The last meal I had was the snack on the plane to Africa. I remembered an apple that I had stuck in my backpack. I quickly fished it out and bit into its crisp skin. I never realized how delicious a simple piece of fruit could be.

I resumed my walk, looking out for anything potentially

edible. I remembered having seen some fruits along the path I walked up yesterday but going back was not an option. The brook soon entered a grove of trees and shrubs. Some were adorned with beautiful flowers, others carried an assortment of unfamiliar fruits. I plucked one that looked like a small brown-skinned pear. It was rather soft and when I squeezed it, it separated into two halves with a large shiny seed in the middle. The smell of the juicy flesh was unfamiliar but quite pleasant. I touched it with my tongue. Sweet, a little tart—it tasted like a mixture of several fruits blended into one, with a new, unfamiliar flavor added to the mix. Could anything this appetizing be dangerous? I bit into it tentatively, letting the juice run down my chin. If this was to kill me, it would still be preferable to starvation.

I plucked another fruit and then three more. The soft fruity texture just slid down into my empty stomach, providing for a moment of inexplicable euphoria. The only drug I had ever experimented with in my youth was marijuana but this was much better. This was truly addictive.

Given the uncertain future of my food supply, I picked a few more of these gifts of nature and stuffed them into my bag.

A short while later I noticed some low bushes along the way that looked quite familiar. They stood less than a foot tall and were covered with small waxy leaves. I squatted to take a closer look. There were many small berries on each branch. Blueberries! A childhood memory suddenly flooded my mind—I could picture the many blueberry bushes in the woods around our house, our long walks to gather them, the sweet smell of blueberry pies and jams my mother used to make. I picked a few excitedly and was about to pop them into my mouth when something stopped me. I examined the berries in my palm more closely. They were dark blue, almost black, with a matte skin, and had a small dimple at the bottom end—exactly the way a blueberry would look. I squeezed one between my fingers, and instead of the juicy flesh I expected to ooze out, I felt a hard pit in the center surrounded by slimy pulp. Disappointed, I chucked them into the bushes and washed my sticky fingers in the clear water of the brook.

A few hours later the countryside changed again. Large boulders started to appear along the path, some large enough to force me to make small detours. Gradually, the easy walk turned into rock climbing as fields of massive boulders were blocking the path. The incline was steep and I had to pause frequently to catch my breath. When I finally reached the ledge, a vast plateau opened up in front of me and the horizon disappeared in a carpet of dense vegetation. I sat down in the shade of a giant tree to rest.

I had no idea where I was or where I was going. I felt like a survivor on a surreal reality show. What was the purpose of all this? Someone had gone through a lot of trouble to get me to Africa—surely not to watch me die. But what was I supposed to do here?

I had no answers to any of my questions. I couldn't even guess. I should have been afraid, but instead I felt a strange equanimity within me that I could not explain. Why was I not scared, alone in an unknown country, without a clear destination and without much hope of returning on my own?

I watched the sun approach the horizon, gradually transforming the surrounding countryside into a dreamlike world of orange, brown, and yellow, growing darker with each passing minute. When only the black silhouettes of the tall cedars and sycamore trees remained visible against the crimson glow, I found a comfortable place on the soft ground and, protected by large boulders on three sides and the now tiny brook on the fourth, lay down to rest.

When I woke up again, the first light was already fringing the impenetrable blackness with a lining of bluish grey. I was lying on my side, my head resting on a grassy knoll. I was facing the gurgling water. Suddenly I felt a strange presence behind me. The surge of adrenalin made me wide awake but I didn't dare to move, just listened intently. There was someone, I was sure.

Then I heard a voice behind my back: "Good morning, my good friend."

I jerked around and found myself staring into the face of a man. He was sitting on the ground just a few feet away from me, his legs crossed under him, his hands folded in his lap. I didn't see the face of the man in my dream last night, but I was sure it was him.

Seeing the panic in my eyes, he raised his palms in a gesture of peace: "Don't be alarmed. I didn't mean to frighten you. Please forgive my intrusion."

I was too startled to respond. He was an older man, perhaps in his fifties or sixties, but he was the type of person whose age was impossible to guess. His facial features were noble, almost aristocratic. He was evoking the image of a Massai warrior, fit for the cover of *National Geographic*. The spear—with a black tear-shaped tip that was resting by his side—only intensified that impression. Yet, he was looking at me with kind, compassionate eyes and a hint of a smile on his lips. There was something inherently non-threatening in his expressions.

I raised myself to a sitting position and we studied each other for a while without speaking. I finally broke the silence. "Are you coming to meet me?"

"Yes," he replied calmly and his smile increased by a small degree.

"Are you taking me somewhere? Why was I just dropped off like this? What's going on?"

"Calm down, my friend," he said. "I am here for you. You are ill—we both know that. But you are ill in more ways than one, in more ways than you realize—"

"What do you mean?" I interrupted. "I have cancer. And I was promised a cure. I don't care what other problems I might have. I am dying of cancer. Nothing else really matters to me right now."

He shook his head, patiently, as if speaking to child. "You are wrong my friend. Everything is connected; everything matters. You have a long way to go and you will need a lot of time."

"But I don't have time," I said. "I was told I had only six months. There is no time to lose. If you are going to help me—" I looked at him questioningly. "Are you a doctor?"

"No," he said and shook his head.

I felt irritation rising in me. "You are not a doctor? You will not try to cure me? So why the hell did you drag me out here. Can you just get me back to the airport? I think I can die more comfortably in my own bed."

He waited for my anger to subside. Then he continued in a calm, reassuring voice: "Please relax and listen. I am not a doctor, not in the sense you understand the term—a doctor of western medicine. I am not even a doctor of eastern medicine, or southern or northern, or holistic, or whatever medicine. The fact of the matter is you don't need a doctor."

He raised his palm to forestall my impending protest. "Patience my friend, please hear me out. There will be plenty of time for questions—tomorrow, next week, next month. You must understand one thing before anything else can make any sense. Are you ready?"

He paused to await my reluctant assent.

"No one can cure you," he continued.

He stopped to let the sentence sink in. But before I could express my disappointment, he resumed.

"The cure is within you—your own body, your own mind."

I listened.

"When your car breaks down, you take it to a mechanic and ask him to fix it. He isolates the problem, adjusts or replaces some parts, and returns it to you in working order, right?"

I nodded.

"But your body is not a car. It is not a machine made from a few interlocking parts that can be adjusted or replaced. If you break a bone then a doctor can fix it and return your body to you in perfect working order. But cancer? A doctor who tries to isolate a complex chronic problem and repair it will fail."

So far this was making sense but what was the solution he was hinting at? I motioned for him to continue.

"Your body is a complex system of interlocking subsystems where any part can impact any other in ways we will never understand. It's like a well-balanced ecosystem. If you start spraying DDT to control mosquitos, you will wipe out hundreds of other species, many of them beneficial, even essential. The collateral damage is worse than the original pest and the ecosystem gets out of balance. Then you will need even deadlier pesticides and there is no end to this cycle."

"Ok, I get it," I said. "Whatever medication I might take will, in the end, make things only worse. So what's the solution?"

"There is no medication for you," he said firmly. "But there is a cure. You will not die here. You will walk out from here stronger than you have even been. You will return home. I promise you that much."

I shook my head. "Tell me how?" I wanted to believe him but could not.

"Follow me," he said. "You have a long way to go."

With that he rose, smoothed out his long, white robe, and using his spear as a hiking stick, picked up the trail along the brook.

"Who are you?" I called after him but he only waved his hand without turning around.

"At least tell me your name," I cried.

He stopped and turned back.

"My name is of no consequence," he said, "just call me X."

"X?" I asked. "Just the letter X? The unknown?"

I tried to get up but could not. My entire body was paralyzed. I tried to call after him again but no sound came out of my throat. He kept walking without looking back. After a few moments he was gone.

'The cure is within you, he had said. I was not sure what to make of these words of wisdom but at some intuitive level, more like a feeling deep down in my stomach, I felt he was right. We have cures, sometimes they work, frequently they don't, and at times they just prolong the agony by a short while. But how could someone simply take control of their own body and influence the course of a deadly disease?

I woke up a few minutes later and rubbed my eyes. What just happened? I looked around. I was alone at the very spot where I lay down last night. The events of the previous two days all came back to me: the ride in the jeep, my endless track through the savannah, the lioness, and the strange man who spoke to me during the night and promised me a cure.

My heart sank at the realization that the promise was just a dream. But it was so unbelievably vivid, so fantastically real.

I sat up, not knowing what to think or do. The sun was just above the horizon and nature started to come alive all around me. I was alone in the middle of nowhere. I took a long drink from the brook, refilled my canteen, and resumed my walk. The man who spoke to me was a dream but his message was real. I felt strangely enlightened and encouraged. The cure is within you, he said. How would I find it?

I resumed my walk along the same brook I had been following the past two days. I sustained my strength by eating the fruits I had found along the way but I began to wonder how long I would be able to survive like that. At least there was an infinite supply of clean, refreshing water. I never knew pure water could taste so good.

As I continued crossing the plateau along the now barely detectable path, reflecting on my last dream, I caught myself talking aloud. The hours of solitude made me argue with myself.

What X said last night made sense. My doctors gave up on me—I had to seek a cure within myself, said one voice.

What are you taking about, said another. There is no X, it's all in your head.

But the idea matters, not who said it, insisted the first.

My body was aching from the long walk, which my sedentary life back home has not prepared me for, but everything else seemed somehow easy and natural. All I had to worry about during the past two days was finding water and nourishment. There were no goals, no milestones, no deadlines, no meetings, or any other minute and mostly annoying obligations that had been the very fabric of my days for most of my adult life. I felt strangely liberated, almost light-headed, at the thought of not having anything to do. If I were to die in six months, I thought with perverted satisfaction, what better way to do it.

When I lay down to sleep that night, I couldn't help wondering if X was going to visit me again. He was my only companion and I hoped he would.

He did wake me up around dawn. He was just there, sitting next to me as he did during the previous night.

"You startled me again," I said, rubbing the sleep out of my eyes.

He only smiled. "It's late. You need to get going."

I rose on my elbow and observed him. His face was furrowed by age and the African sun. I wasn't sure if he was smiling or if the placid expression was a permanent feature of his being.

"Where are we going anyway?" I asked to continue the conversation.

"Your new home."

"My new home?" I repeated incredulously. "I thought I was going to some hospital or sanatorium."

He cut me off with a resolute sweep of his hand. "You already are in the best sanatorium. Just look around." He paused while scanning the gradually whitening horizon. "There is no better place for you, no place more natural, more conducive to healing.

"That's great but I don't need a vacation," I said. "I need a doctor or a healer or a shaman or whatever—"

He again silenced my protest.

"You don't need any wise men; you are your own best healer."

I looked at him in disbelief. "What exactly do you want me

to do? I know nothing of medicine. What would be my first step?"

"Well, there are certain steps to take and certain milestones to reach."

"Ah," I sighed with relief.

"But I say this only for the benefit of your western mind. You have been brought up in an environment where everything must have its proper place, everything must be analyzed, categorized, divided and subdivided, and where every action must have a beginning and an end, with a series of intermediate steps to be followed."

"Exactly. That's what scientific medicine is about."

"Your medicine, perhaps. But your medicine gave up on you, remember? It failed to subdivide your body into independent compartments that could be attacked in isolation. It can't be done."

"Ok, ok," I said in resignation. "But you said there were some steps or whatever for me to take."

"If it helps you to think in terms of steps, then steps there will be."

"Good. Now we are getting somewhere. So what's my first step? I need to get started. Now."

He smiled at my exuberance. "I have some good news for you, my friend," and when I didn't answer, he completed his pronouncement: "You have already passed your first step."

I began to suspect what he was going to tell me but let him proceed with his lecture.

"Your first step—perhaps the most important one of all— you have taken back home, when you decided to follow my invitation. You could have just given up. Your physicians gave you six months and said there was nothing they could do. Why did you not accept their verdict? Why have you decided to take a chance on an anonymous phone call?"

"Why?" I asked in return.

"Because you were not ready to die. Deep down in yourself, in places you didn't even know existed, you knew the doctors were wrong. And you decided—against all rational thought—

to follow this feeling, this instinct buried deep inside you. That was your first step toward reclaiming your health."

He fell silent and I could not think of a suitable reply, not even a suitable objection. He was right; what I did was irrational, bordering on insanity, but I did it anyway. I was here, in the middle of Africa, lying beside a man I knew nothing about. But it felt all right.

He rose to continue the walk, and just like last night I was unable to follow him.

When I woke up, I realized it was again a dream. I was alone and I felt deeply confused. I kept following an illusion produced by my own brain. But the arguments—they all sounded rational.

I rose, ate some of the fruit I still had left from yesterday and refilled my bottle from the brook. Then I set out to continue my walk, not knowing where I was going. I was not ready to roll over and die, X had said. That much was true.

I walked slowly, letting my mind wander and try to sort out all the conflicting thoughts and messages that were eddying around my head. But there was no turning back, that much I knew.

So what should be my next step? I decided to ask X, should he visit me again.

The sun was already setting when I noticed the silhouette of some dwelling in the distance. As I came closer, I discovered it was a small round hut. The walls were made of dried reddish adobe. The two openings on each side that served as windows were barred by interlaced tree branches anchored in the clay. The door, woven from thicker branches and tied together with leather straps was hung on two hinges, also made of leather. This simple construction was covered by a roof of dried palm fronds interwoven into a gradually rising spiral.

"Hello," I said cautiously. "Is anyone there?"

There was no reply and so I pushed aside the simple latch holding the door in place. I had to bow my head to pass under the low doorframe into the semi-darkness of the hut. There was only a single room, lit by the almost horizontal rays of the setting sun coming in through one of the barred windows. The furnishings consisted of a rough mattress resting on wooden supports close to the rounded wall and a simple shelf containing a few cooking utensils. A long spear with a black tear-shaped tip, almost identical to the one carried by X, and a long knife were suspended from wooden pegs sunken into the wall.

My new home?

There was not much more to discover inside so I stepped out again. I walked around to the back of the hut where, to my great surprise, I discovered a small pen with several live chickens. In the adjacent large enclosure was a pair of goats, both completely black. One of them raised her head to examine me as I passed by but quickly returned to her previous occupation of chewing the tough brown grass on the other side of the wooden fence. Further down were several cultivated plots containing various plants. I pulled one out—it was some kind of a sweet potato, perhaps a yam? Another was a type of a small yellow squash. I did not recognize anything else.

My biggest worry now was water. The path I had been following up the plateau had deviated from the brook a few hours ago. My canteen was almost empty and there was no sign of any well or other water source around the hut.

I noticed a barely visible trail leading away from the hut. Despite the impending darkness, I decided to follow it for a while. Just a few minutes into my walk, I heard something that sounded like running water. I broke into a trot and when I reached the low ridge forming the horizon, I saw a stream of water rushing over large granite boulders. It was much wider than the brook.

In my rush to explore, I forgot to bring my water bottle. I kneeled down and using my cupped hands, filled my stomach with the crystalline liquid. Delicious.

I returned to the hut, this time walking slowly and observing all that was growing along the path. The interior of the hut was already dark when I entered. I did not recall having seen any lantern and, even if I had, I would not have been able to light it. Barely recognizing the contours of the hut's interior, I put out my hand and sliding it along the wall tested my way to where I remembered seeing the cot. I lay down. The night was pleasantly warm, there was no need for a blanket. I listened to the evocative noises coming in from the darkness outside.

When I turned to my side, X was seated next to me.

"Welcome to your new home," he said. "I hope you have found everything to your satisfaction."

I glanced at my nightly companion. "It's all right," I said. "But what's next?"

"Your next step, hmm—" he seemed to contemplate the problem. Was he just making it up as we went along?

"You have already discovered on your own what the next step is," he continued his thought, "and have made good progress towards completing it."

"How so?" I said.

"You began to recognize your unique relationship with your surroundings." He seemed to be searching for the right words to convey his message. "Try to reflect on what went through your mind during the past two days. You were dropped off with no possessions other than the clothes on your back in the middle of an unknown forest. Think: What did you need to survive two lonely days?"

I just shrugged, not knowing where he was going with his thought. He answered his question for me: "All you needed was water to drink, something to eat, and a place to rest. Am I right?" Since I did not volunteer any comments, he continued. "You drank only water. Was it not the best tasting thirst quencher you have had in years?"

I had to admit: slurping up the cool water from the brook using my cupped hand after several hours of walking was a delight.

"As for nourishment," he continued, "you sampled not

only bananas but also mkobe, kwa-ra, nyada, ..."

"If you say so—I really had no idea what I was eating."

"But that's my point," he said with obvious delight. "You had never seen these fruits before. Yet you ate them and they sustained you for two days. How did you know what to eat? Think of an alien from another planet—could he do that? Or would he have attempted to eat leaves or tree bark or rocks? Why didn't you? Your instincts told you. They told you what tastes good, which is exactly what your body needed."

"Isn't that pretty obvious?" I protested.

"No. Remember the nili-jaa you almost ate but, luckily, chose not to?"

"What nili? Do you mean those strange-looking blueberries?"

"Yes," he confirmed. "That berry is called nili-jaa. Had you swallowed it, you would still be in serious pain right now. A few more and we would not be talking at all."

I felt anger rising in me. "You almost let me poison myself? Without any warning?"

"Look," he said patiently. "You picked it up, examined it, intended to eat it—but you didn't. Why?"

"It just did not look right. That's why."

"Yet you have never seen it before, have you?" He looked at me triumphantly. "You have never seen it, it actually looked deceptively similar to a blueberry, yet something made you reject it. That something saved your life—or at least some nasty stomach cramps. What was that something?" He paused for me to reflect.

What he said was right yet I could not explain it.

"Does this have anything to do with my next step?" I asked.

"Everything." He nodded. "People have been roaming these plains and forests for millennia in search of food and, in doing so, have developed many instincts that helped them survive. The few thousand years of civilization have not erased our instincts—they are still with us, perhaps a bit dormant, but they are there. Your next step was to re-awaken them. Reclaim these precious gifts of our forefathers and let them serve you as an invisible hand, guiding and protecting you as you go through life. You have already started doing it—something you could have never accomplished while surrounded by concrete, glass, and plastic. For that you had to come here and be forced to rely on yourself for survival from one moment to the next. Learn to listen to the subtle cues your body is sending you every second. It knows exactly what it needs. All you have to do is follow."

What he said began to make a lot sense and I felt empowered by my new insights.

"If waking up an ancient dormant instinct was my last accomplishment, what's next?"

"I am sorry my friend," he replied, "but that's something I can't really tell you."

"What do you mean?" I asked incredulously. "You can't tell me what my next step should be? Then how will I know what to do?"

"That you will have to discover for yourself. It is an essential part of the process. I am not a doctor and I do not prescribe anything—medicines, diets, therapies—nothing. And you cannot be a passive follower. The doctor-please-fix-me approach simply does not work. Remember what I told you earlier: the cure is within you. What you need to do is discover each new step on your own, just like you discovered the preceding ones. After all, it was you who decided to come here and it is you who is now beginning to discover how perfectly suited your body and your mind are to surviving in this environment. Trust yourself and the next step will become as obvious as the next sunrise."

I made another feeble attempt to pry out additional information from X. "Tell me at least how many steps there are in this process?"

X poked me in the chest with his forefinger. "You need to work on undoing your western indoctrination, your obsessions with precise categorizations, dissections, serializations. You think that every step must have a beginning and an ending, and that each step starts wherever the previous one ends. But nature is never that orderly. Just think of your last step. When do you expect to have recovered all your ancestral instincts? Probably never. This task will occupy the rest of your life, however long it may be. As you go on living, you will be continuously gaining new insights into life. They will start emerging seemingly out of nowhere, one after another, and soon you will be able to weave them into a stream of astuteness—a deep, almost subconscious understanding of the world around you and your place within it."

When I woke up, it took me a while to recall where I was. I was lying on my side, staring into a coarse ochre-colored mud wall. I rolled over on my back, slowly recognizing the palm thatch above me and recalling the events of the preceding two days. The room was empty. The sunrays falling in through the window above me painted a barred rectangle of light on the opposite wall. I felt rested but the feeling of hunger nagging in my empty stomach soon brought me face to face with reality. I recalled my last dialog with X. My hunger instinct was clearly very much alive.

I realized that I had never experienced real hunger before. People say they are starving when they have not eaten a big meal in a few hours. But real hunger? Try to eat nothing but unfamiliar fruit for three days and you will experience what real hunger feels like—a carnal urge commanding you to get up and do something about it. And do it now!

Back home, in my comfort-minded society, there was no easy way to get really hungry. I had never been in a situation where I could not have opened a fridge filled with who-knows-what. And should that fail, a fast-food restaurant or a convenience store, open 24-7, was always a few minutes away. I would have had to go out of my way—get lost while hiking in the wilderness—to end up fasting for more than a few hours.

Another urgent growl in my stomach rudely interrupted my philosophizing. I could have killed for a plate of pancakes bathed in maple syrup, eggs sunny-side up, and crispy strips of bacon—not to mention a cup of strong coffee. I heaved myself up from the cot, stretched my back—aching from the travails of the previous days—and walked across the room to give the utility shelves a more careful inspection. A couple of kettles of different sizes, a dull knife, some type of a ladle carved out of wood, an oil lamp—too bad I hadn't noticed it last night.

I lifted a piece of colorful woven cloth that was covering a small wicker basket. To my great delight, it contained several pieces of bread, the type I used to see in the Middle-eastern stores back home: flat, unleavened, sprinkled with sesame and linseeds. I grabbed a piece and hungrily tore off a bite with my teeth. It was chewy, but full of flavor. I wolfed it down with two more bites and went for another piece. Only with the third piece did I manage to slow down, letting the firm texture dissolve in my mouth before swallowing it. This was clearly the greatest delicacy I had ever tasted in my life.

Having staved off my starvation, I waked out the door to re-examine my new surroundings. The fact that X only kept me company at night was annoying. I felt like Robinson Crusoe and having my Friday around at daytime would be useful.

The bread was a nice compliment and I was eternally grateful to whoever thought of providing me with it—but what about the next meal? Or something tastier, like that bacon I was hallucinating about earlier? Where did bacon come from anyway? I had never consciously thought of pigs when enjoying crunchy strips of bacon on my cheese-bacon-burger.

I had not noticed any pigs around my property—domestic or wild—and even if I had, there was no way I could have turned one into bacon. I appraised the spear hanging on the wall above the bed. This was the first serious weapon I had ever held in my hands and I was sure that I would not be able to thrust it through a frantically oinking animal. How easy for city people to come home moaning: I'm so hungry, I could kill for a double burger! I wished they were here now, to face the inconvenient fact that the juicy meat patty was just recently a part of a breathing animal, which they didn't have to kill. Someone else in some anonymous slaughter house did it, thus erasing all unpleasant connections between food and death.

The fact that I had never killed an animal larger than a housefly in my entire life had become painfully apparent. I had to overcome that inhibition if I wanted to eat some meat, but the vision of killing a lamb for a lamb chop was too raw. My head began to spin and I began to feel queasy. I had to sit down for a minute.

Would a smaller animal, something lower on the food chain, be easier to handle—not just physically but also emotionally? I fixed my eyes on one of the chickens strutting around and clucking restlessly while looking for seeds in the brown grass. Could I handle that? With the machete perhaps? Just one swipe across the neck. But people often talk about running around like a chicken with its head cut off. The image of a headless chicken spurting blood made me sick. Maybe some other day. At this point, I was ready to turn vegetarian.

As I walked past the pen, I disturbed one of the hens that was resting in a corner in what looked like a heap of dried grass. It got up reluctantly to keep a safe distance and at that moment I realized that she was sitting on a nest. I counted nine brown eggs nicely arranged in a circle where the hen had been sitting. Until now I had seen eggs only in their neat break-resistant packages by the dozen, never in a messy nest under a bird.

I picked up four of them and took them back to the hut, not having a real plan for what to do with them. I knew how to boil or fry an egg—on a gas stove. I needed fire but that would take too long and I was just too hungry. The vision of Rocky Balboa breaking a dozen eggs into a glass and drinking them raw before running out to train came back to me. Reluctantly, I broke one of the eggs into a bowl. I smelled it. Not great. I broke the remaining eggs, blended them with a wooden fork into a uniform liquid, and lifted the bowl to my lips. I had never tasted raw eggs before. The slippery texture was surprising. I tilted my head back and let the entire content of the bowl slide down my throat in three big gulps. I wiped my mouth with the back of my hand and remained standing for a moment to process the experience. My hunger was gone.

The rest of the day I spent exploring my surroundings. My hut was standing on a low plateau with sparse vegetation. The river made a loop at its base, protecting it on three sides like the moat of a medieval castle. The gentle slopes on both banks were full of lush vegetation, including many of the fruit trees I learned to know when coming up the path. I also saw many varieties of birds, lizards, and insects. I found a shallow spot in the river and waded to the other bank. I continued walking for a while but the landscape was an endless repetition of rolling hills and shallow green valleys.

When I returned home, it was already getting dark and I was exhausted. I finished the last piece of by now very dry bread from my welcome basket and fell asleep as soon as I lay down.

When I opened my eyes, X was again sitting next to me, placid and observant.

"I see that you managed to prevent a few chicks from hatching," he said.

I looked at the heap of egg shells that I didn't bother to throw away yesterday.

"I was starving," I said, not knowing if I should feel guilty or proud.

"You are making good progress."

I raised myself on one elbow to better read his face. "What progress?"

"Major progress. You are working on your next step—one of the most important ones for people like you," he added gravely.

"Drinking raw eggs is part of my cure?" I asked incredulously. "And what exactly do you mean by people like me?"

"No, not eggs," he said. He crossed his legs under him and laid his spear on the ground to get more comfortable. "I am not going to prescribe any diets for you. No, absolutely no diets. That's how you westerners like to think: Doctor, please fix me. Give me something that will make me whole again. If you broke your arm, I might do that. If the lioness took a bite out of you, I would try to heal you. But cancer is not an accident and there is no prescription that will fix it. I already told you: You need to do it yourself."

"I am hearing your message," I said with some impatience, "but I still don't see the path."

"You need to change," he said. "Change everything about your lifestyle."

"So this isn't enough of a lifestyle change?" I gestured dramatically, pointing to my surroundings.

He shook his head resolutely. We sat quietly for a long time, I trying to process the message I had just been given, and X waiting patiently for me to react. I was confused and conflicting thoughts were racing through my mind. I had always considered the developments of the past few centuries as great and welcome progress—tools and machines that made our lives easier, air-conditioned and heated homes, hot and cold water coming out of every faucet, a cornucopia of foods from all parts of the world, medical breakthroughs eradicating pests and diseases—but all this was now being questioned as desirable. Was this explosive progress making us sick? And if so, was it then worth it?

When I woke up, I was very confused. There was a realization growing in me that I had to make many changes in my life, but what specifically? And how long would this take?

I tried to remember how many days I had already been away from civilization. The fact that I had to reconstruct it from what I had been doing every day scared me. I decided to keep a calendar. It would help me maintain at least a tenuous connection with the world I had left behind. More importantly, I wanted to know when the six months my doctor gave me to live would be up.

Not having brought any paper or pens with me, I considered various alternatives. I could cut notches into some branch or trunk of a tree, but I preferred to keep the calendar indoors. Cutting notches into the door or window frames did not seem too practical since there was not much wood to work with. I also considered tying knots into strings or gathering pebbles in different containers but none of this seemed convenient. In the end, I decided to use the charcoal from the fire to make marks on the wall. One mark for each day arranged in groups of seven; each month starting with a new row. This simple scheme turned out to be sufficiently visual to follow the passage of time. I sat on the bed, considering the four black marks. How many more would I be able to make?

I needed some time to think. I got up and just started walking without having any specific destination in mind. I walked past the corral, followed the narrow path down to the river, then continued upstream for an hour or two—time did not seem to mean much.

I reached a bend in the stream where the water had carved out a deep lagoon. I sat down to rest, watching the water ripple by lazily. I noticed a few fish darting around and recalled a time when my dad used to take me fishing. I remembered being bored to death, waiting for hours for any fish to bite, and listening to Dad's explanations as to why fishing was the most natural occupation a man could indulge in.

I should try it now, I thought. Killing a fish with my own hands seemed a lot less traumatic than having to butcher a mammal or even a dumb bird. But how would I catch one? I needed to ask X if he had any fish hooks but I suspected he would tell me to make one myself.

Perhaps I could catch it with my bare hands? I have seen it done—in movies.

In a bout of excitement, I took off my shoes and waded into the stream. The fish seemed unimpressed but skillfully maintained a safe distance. I attempted to drive them into the shallow area of the bend but they were too smart for that.

I gave up, frustrated. But now I was more determined than ever. It was a personal challenge: man against nature, intellect over instinct.

On my way home, and pretty much the rest of the day, I kept thinking about all the possible ways one could devise to get a fish out of the water.

As soon as X showed up that night, I asked him what my next step would be.

"Give your body what it was designed to consume," he said.

"I think my body was designed to consume some fish right now."

X laughed. "What's stopping you?"

"Their instincts," I said annoyed. "They don't like to be eaten."

X laughed again. "Outsmarting smart fish is a nice challenge. If you succeed, you can eat as many as you like."

"So eating fish is good for me?"

"If your body tells you to eat fish, then eat fish. Your body knows best."

"And if my body tells me to eat a gallon of ice cream?"

"How do you propose making it out here?"

I realized the absurdity of my request but was still not convinced. "So how do I really know what to eat? Are you not going to tell me about proper nutrition, vitamins, minerals, that sort of thing?"

"No," he said resolutely. "You can eat whatever you like."

I looked at him skeptically. "That's a good diet. Why didn't my doctor tell me that?"

"I like your sense of humor," X said, "but things are much simpler than you think. Your doctor can't tell you to eat whatever you like because your world is full of crap. But look around here." He let his hand sweep the horizon in a grand circle. "Whatever you find here will be good for you. If you only use this grocery store and your instincts, you can't go wrong."

I was less than thrilled with what he was telling me.

"So basically I have to live on berries, beetles, and raw meat, is that it?" I asked, feeling a strong bite of indignation in my chest.

"Not at all." X held up his palms in a conciliatory gesture. "You don't have to return to prehistory. Fire, for example, is a very useful invention."

"Indeed." I nodded emphatically. "I noticed some matches in the hut so I won't have to reinvent fire."

X ignored my sarcasm. "Our bodies are well adapted to cooked food, wouldn't you agree?"

I agreed enthusiastically.

"In fact, cooking is what made us human, did you know that? Apes spend most of their day chewing on leaves, fruits, or whatever raw food they can find just to stay alive. Supporting a large energy-hungry brain like ours needs more nutrition, much more than what you could get from raw food."

I nodded in agreement. "I know that. Cooking was our ticket to intelligence, culture, and a total domination of the planet."

"Yes. But also to junk food and lazy living. But don't worry, there is no need to wind the clock back all the way to the dawn of humanity. You only need to undo a few thousand years—that brief period of time during which the pace of progress was too explosive for our bodies to adapt."

"So if I hear you right, my next step is to—"

"To put your body in harmony with the environment for which it was designed," he finished my sentence.

I could think of no more objections as he delivered his final conclusion: "That's why you are here. This environment deprives you of all the bad things that civilization has given you. You are down to the bare essentials of life; you are now a hunter, a gatherer, and an early farmer. Now, try to go fishing."

As soon as I woke up and hastily drank a glass of mango juice, I packed a couple of bananas and a mango into my bag and returned to the river. I still had no idea how to get the fish without any tackle, but I was determined more than ever to solve the problem. I remembered a *National Geographic* special, showing men in some African country building fish traps. These were large cages, woven out of sticks and vines, having a funnel-like opening for an easy entry but an almost impossible escape. The idea was sound but when I looked around, I had no idea where to begin.

I decided to build a dam across the stream, hoping to prevent an easy escape downstream. I took off my pants and my shirt and started to gather heavy boulders, placing them in a line across the stream. It was heavy work and I had to splash myself constantly to keep cool. I then dropped smaller rocks in between the large ones to close any major gaps. The water was still getting through, it even rose a little behind the dam, but the fish couldn't pass it.

I straightened up from the heavy work and admired my construction for a moment. I broke off two leafy branches from a tree, walked a few steps upstream, and beating the water with one branch in each outstretched arm, drove the fish toward the barrier. The fish obeyed but at the last second each took a sharp tack to one side and darted past me into the safety of open water. I tried my luck a few more times, with the same outcome.

I sat down in the shade of a tree. It was frustrating to think that all that hard labor was in vain—a mere demonstration of how naive and helpless a city dweller can be.

I decided to make one more attempt before giving up all hope. I used the same branches as before to herd my school of fish toward the dam but this time kept them close to the shore. When they were ready to turn and dart back, I quickly veered to the side and pushed them toward a shallow sand bank near the shore. There were at least two dozen fish in front of me and most managed to shoot past me before the water got too shallow. But one panicked, tried a quick left turn and then a right again, but each time I managed to scare it back with my branches. Having no way of retreating, it tried to wiggle over a submerged sand bar. For a fraction of a second it got stuck on top of it, thrashing frantically to free itself, but this tiny miscalculation slowed it down sufficiently for me to leap toward it. With my cupped hands, I scooped it up and propelled it out of the water. It landed on the grassy bank, far enough from the water. It began to thrash violently in futile attempts to reach the safety of the water's edge. I watched with startled satisfaction as its jumps became less frequent and less powerful. After a few moments, it just lay there, exhausted, flapping its tail fin against the grass as life continued to dissipate from its shiny, sleek body.

I kept watching it long after all movement had ceased, my heart still beating hard with the excitement of the hunt. When I calmed down, I took it back to the hut and using my knife, cleaned it as best as I still remembered from the days on the water with my father so many years ago. I impaled it on a long stick and fried it over the open fire. It was tiny, more suitable for a home aquarium than a plate, but it tasted better than anything I had eaten in a long time.

I recounted my adventure to X with undisguised pride.

"I am glad you enjoyed it," he said. "It was good for you— both the hunt and the meal."

"There is something I need to ask you," I said. "Back home, I could have eaten a nice little fish like this any time. Why have I usually chosen some junk food instead?"

Since X didn't answer right away, I proceeded to explain the dilemma I had been considering for a while now.

"Call it nature, instincts, whatever, but there is something in every living being that subconsciously tells it what to do and what to avoid to survive and to procreate," I said. "A sheep, no matter how thirsty, won't drink sea water because it would make it sick. A wolf will not eat grass or tree bark, because it cannot digest them. No animal in the wild will consume anything that's bad for its health, am I right?"

X nodded in agreement, waiting for me to pose my question.

"Why do people then eat and drink junk, even though we

know it's bad for us? Has something gone wrong in our evolution that disabled the natural instincts that protect all other living organisms from hurting themselves—knowingly and willingly?"

X nodded gravely.

"It is our own intelligence that carries most of the blame," he said.

"Sounds paradoxical."

"Not if you think about it more deeply. There are two reasons for this, both related to our intelligence. The first is our uncanny ability to produce unnatural foods."

"Unnatural—meaning synthetic?"

"Not even that. It may be foods that do occur in nature but only in minute quantities."

"Like caffeine? Or alcohol?" I asked.

"Exactly. In fact, you may have noticed a number of coffee plants growing in the neighborhood and there is certainly plenty of fruit and grains to make moonshine. Should I be worried? Hardly. You have no idea how far away you are from a liquor store or a Starbucks Café—both literally and figuratively."

"Fine, I won't turn into an addict here but what's wrong with all the other stuff I could get at my supermarket? What's wrong with bread?"

"The problem is that almost nothing you will find there has been left in its original state. Everything has been processed, altered, upgraded—it is pretty much man-made. Flower is made by milling grains and removing the surrounding shells—but those contain exactly the important fibers that help your digestion. Fats are made by solidifying oils using the magic of hydrogenation. This makes saturated fats—bad stuff that people were not designed to eat. Chocolate—everyone knows that this is sin-food. Not that pure cocoa is bad for you, but the fat and sugar more than make up for it."

"But the body needs some sugar and fat. Isn't that exactly why we crave these?"

"True, but neither pure fat nor sugar occur freely in nature;

they must be extracted from other foods. When you eat only unprocessed fruits, vegies, and grains, it is impossible to consume in a single meal the same amount of fat and sugar contained in even a single donut."

It all began to sound very plausible. The body knew exactly what it needed but we have tricked it by altering the environment from which it was satisfying its needs.

Then I remembered what he had said earlier. "What's the second reason for our bad eating habits?"

"This has to do with food's connection to culture," he resumed his lecture. "Animals eat simply because they are hungry. People have elevated eating from a necessity to a social event. We often eat because of emotions rather than hunger. We eat because we feel happy or sad, depressed or excited, frustrated or bored, or just for the sheer pleasure of it."

"Animals don't do that," I agreed.

"That's because it's an acquired behavior. It has been transmitted to us from our parents and grandparents. It needs verbal communication. There is no species other than humans where parents can force their young to eat anything. To do that, the young needs to understand the concept of punishment: Finish your plate or else!"

"I have never been forced to eat anything," I remembered, "but if I didn't, there was no dessert."

"That's one and the same—sticks or carrots—no pun intended. Your eating habits are being manipulated by people who think they know better. The promise of a dessert elevates fats and sugars to the most desirable part of the meal and degrades the rest to punishment. Years of persistent pressure destroyed your body's inborn instincts of what it really needs. Food becomes a reward. Then for the rest of your life you use food to celebrate successes, or to remedy stress, or to console yourself in tough situations."

When I woke up, the memory of my fish hunt resurfaced as if recalling a favorite sitcom episode. It was fun, but it was also exhausting. I may have expended more calories in catching the little fish than it had given me. There had to be a better way to get at this precious protein.

I revisited the idea of fish traps and fish hooks, but couldn't conjure any practical solution. Then I remembered spear fishing. Many years ago I went on a diving trip in the Caribbean. I was given a harpoon propelled by a coiled spring, and I even managed to harm a few fish.

The idea got me excited. I had no way of making a harpoon, but I could make some kind of a spear. I took my knife and walked out toward the bushes. Most trees were either too thick, too gnarly, or too crooked. After a long search I found what I was looking for: A young tree with a long, slender trunk of about an inch in diameter. I cut it down at the base. Then I removed all its branches except for one almost at the tip of the trunk. I cut it to the same length as the top of the trunk, thus forming a kind of a fork. I sharpened both points and carved them into inward facing barbed hooks.

I hefted the new weapon in my arm. It felt light and dangerous. I walked toward the river using my new spear as a walking stick. The sun was reflecting brilliantly in the millions of little ripples of the stream. I kicked off my shoes and carefully waded in. I spotted a few fish but they were darting by too quickly. Gradually, I made my way toward the bend where the water was flowing slowly and the surface was smooth. I spotted several fish staying still in the slowly moving current. In slow motion I advanced toward them, holding the spear at the ready. I felt my heart beating as I took aim at the closest one. I lowered the spear until the tips almost touched the water's surface, then thrust it forward. I was fast enough, but the spear missed its target and the fish just darted away.

I made another attempt a few minutes later, with the same result. How could I have missed? The spear tip was a mere foot away.

Then I remembered a long-forgotten lesson from high school, something about refraction. Light bends when it enters water and so objects appear to be somewhere else. But where? Closer? Farther? I dipped the spear into the water: It seemed to be bent at the water's surface, pointing downward. I had to aim lower, closer to me, to hit the target. I snuck up on another large fish, aimed a few inches below where I saw it, and thrust the spear in. I felt the tip making contact with something and at that same instant it started to jerk around violently. I had to use both hands to lift it out of the water. Stuck between the two barbed tips was a beautiful fish, fighting desperately for its life. I hoisted it into the air to make sure it couldn't fall off and waded back to shore, where I ended its struggle with my knife.

I could not wait to share my experiences of the day with X.

"I see that you managed to secure a steady supply of healthy protein," he said as soon as he sat down.

"The fish here are delicious," I agreed. "When I remember what I used to eat back home, I shudder. But why did you have to drag me out to Africa to show me that? You could have just told me what to eat and I am sure I could have found the same stuff at the supermarket."

He shook his head. "Would you have believed me? Would you have blindly followed my instructions?"

I shrugged with little conviction.

"Exactly. Back home I had no control over you. Here you don't have a choice. You will have to use the same weapon— your intelligence, which taught you bad eating habits—to reverse the trend. You will have to use your ingenuity to survive. Nature will repay you by resetting your mind and restoring your body to what it was designed to do."

Seeing the skeptical look on my face, he asked: "Have you ever been on a diet?"

"Not really," I admitted truthfully. "Once I tried to lose a few pounds. Not for any health reasons but to impress a woman I was dating. And I did succeed—lost some five, six pounds in a few weeks."

"And?"

"The fling ended, I kissed my diet goodbye along with the girlfriend, and in less than a month I was right back where I started, even gained a few extra pounds."

"What you just described is a classic scenario of a dieter," X said. "Diets never work. Period. And why not, you should be asking."

"Why not?"

"Two reasons. First, it is impossible to lose the pounds that took many months or years to accumulate in just a few short weeks. You can shed a few pounds, mostly water, but then your body panics. It goes into a state of self-preservation, it slows down the metabolism, it refuses to give up any of its accumulated fat reserves."

I nodded in agreement. "And the second reason?"

"The second reason is even more important. It is the sheer frustration of food deprivation—you are simply not allowed to eat anything you like. This, combined with the excruciatingly slow progress of weight-loss, generally breaks the spirit of even the most determined person. Luckily for you, this can't happen here. There is no fridge to dive into to console yourself, no supermarket to reward yourself with treats and junk. This environment will reprogram your mind whether you like it or not."

"But why are we talking about weight loss anyway? I'm dying of cancer," I objected.

"I know, but in nature, everything is connected. If you abuse your body and don't give it what it needs, you may grow fat or you may become ill, or you may grow fat first and then become ill. The cause is the same, only the symptoms are different."

"So you propose to cure me by starvation."

X rolled his eyes. "I think you are trying to be difficult but my patience is infinite. Listen and pay close attention. There will be no food deprivation. On the contrary, I want you to eat well and I want you to eat whatever you like."

"Isn't that a contradiction in terms?" I said.

"Not out here. You may feel like eating a double cheeseburger but it can't happen, so you learn to appreciate the taste of the fish you just caught. Gradually, your taste will shift. Eventually, whatever you crave and whatever is good for you will become the same."

He raised his palm to stifle my impending protest. "Taste is largely acquired. Look at coffee. It has no nutritional value, caffeine is a poison, yet millions of people simply need it. They need it to survive, they say, and they mean it. Where does this unstoppable urge come from? Children don't like the taste or even the smell of coffee. They wonder how anyone can drink that stuff. But with time, repeated exposure, and lots of sugar and cream added, one gradually develops the taste for it."

"But that's a contrived example," I protested. "Caffeine is a drug; it is addictive. What does it have to do with real food? Are you suggesting that I had to develop the taste for cheese and that I would not like it otherwise?"

"Surprisingly, yes. Just compare cheese and tofu. Most westerners love cheese but very few like tofu. Many find any type of bean curd outright revolting. Yet there isn't a single person in Asia who does not love tofu, yet few are crazy about any kind of cheese. Spoiled milk, they say, stinky and outright revolting. Why these differences? Asians and Caucasians are not different species. We all have the same physiology. The only reason is exposure. It simply takes time to acquire the taste for many foods."

"I actually like tofu," I said almost dreamily. I closed my eyes and imagined myself in my favorite Japanese restaurant.

"Will I ever go back home?" I asked.

X only nodded.

"Suppose I really do. Won't I naturally revert to the same bad habits, the same old foods, and get sick again?"

X thought for a while before launching into a long explanation.

"The problem is that a diet always has a beginning and an ending. It is automatically perceived as a period of suffering and self-sacrifice, and so it leads to an even greater desire for the forbidden foods. It is human nature that forbidding something only increases the desire for it. The proverbial forbidden fruit, which is not a fruit at all, but excess sugar and fat, is why it is so hard to stay on a planned diet.

"Out here there are no specific limitations and no forbidden foods. After a while, you will have reprogrammed your mind and be free from any desires for the unhealthy foods you used to like. You will start to like your new types of food and stop craving those you can't have. You will start feeling great, have more energy, and this feedback loop will erase any dormant desires for your old junk food.

"Eventually, you will be able to say that you don't care for french fries and actually mean it. Getting to this stage takes time but once you reach it, you will be able to go home. You will feel a complete sense of freedom, a freedom of choice, where you are no longer a slave of your eating habits and food desires."

I was still unconvinced that people could not make this transition back home.

"It is possible to achieve that at home," X consented, "but it is a long process full of pitfalls. No one goes from a food junkie to a health nut overnight. If you attempt to break your bad habits by force, your body will rebel and you will quickly end up where you started. The transformation needs to happen gradually, in stages, and at each stage you are in danger of failing.

"At the start, you are simply in denial—you feel that your eating habits are perfectly fine and there is no need to do anything. At some point you reach a stage of contemplation, and you begin to wonder if some minor adjustments wouldn't ameliorate your weight gain or perhaps some minor health issues. At that stage you are ready to take some concrete actions toward your goals, but the most critical phase is what follows your initial steps—you need to sustain the effort in the long run and this is where doubts creep in and relapses happen.

"You do not have enough time to go through this long and perilous process of gradual lifestyle change. You need to do this now and you cannot afford to fail. This is why you are here."

When I woke up, I thought about this long conversation with X. I knew it was just another dream but where did all the insights, the arguments, the conclusions, and the counterexamples come from? In a conscious state, I knew little about the subject. In my dreams, perhaps conditioned by my new experiences, I must have been reaching deep down into areas of subconscious domains that in the past have been masked by the pressures of civilization.

***

As the days passed, I lost all fear of my surroundings and was keen to discover new areas father away from my hut. Each day of exploring yielded gifts of new fruits, berries, and tubers, which I experimented with in my primitive kitchen.

Other than the occasional fish I managed to spear, the eggs from my hens, and the goat milk, my diet became mostly vegan. At first I was worried about eating so many raw fruits and vegetables every day. I expected the usual bouts of heartburn, indigestion, or gas, which at home I managed to keep under control using various antacids and other medications. But none of these annoying symptoms had materialized here. I found that pleasantly surprising but most puzzling.

X delivered an explanation the following evening.

"It is quite ironic that many people avoid the healthiest of foods because of the way they feel afterwards. The sad truth is that, while digestive discomforts may occur when eating fruits or vegetables, it is really the fatty and unbalanced foods in the background that are the real culprits."

I didn't see the connection and waited for X's further explanation.

"You see, when you eat a lot of fatty junk every day for years and years, your digestive system learns what to expect with each meal—and, sadly, it adapts to it by producing large amounts of acidic stomach juices to digest all the fat. When you then eat an occasional orange, more acid is added to the mix and the stomach rebels by heartburn or other digestive discomforts."

"But I never experienced any problems when I was young," I objected, "even though my eating habits were abominable."

"At a young age," X continued, "your body can adapt to just about any type of abuse and achieve some semblance of balance. With advancing age, you don't get as much discretion any longer. Your digestive system has been overused and can no longer work adequately. The consequence of this unbalanced, unhealthy, and unnatural type of eating is the increased need for medication to keep digestion under control."

I accepted this explanation with great relief, knowing that the nearest pharmacy was hundreds of miles away.

"But there is more," X continued. "Replacing fat with complex carbohydrates—fruits, vegies, beans, grains, and such—is doubly beneficial. Not only is there much less fat to digest but since fruits contain natural acids, they help your body to digest whatever fat there is remaining."

"Interesting," I had to admit. "So eating fruits and vegies does not burden my stomach."

"On the contrary," X concluded. "It spares it much effort and so it will function properly, free of medication and free of any health problems for your entire life."

My only hope was that this would be much longer than the few months my doctor had granted me.

***

I was barely aware of the passage of time. Each day transitioned into the same peaceful night full of enchanting sounds, and each morning's sunrise spurred me into action to take care of my food and other daily necessities.

I continued maintaining my calendar by adding a new bar just before going to sleep. I was now looking at five complete rows, with a sixth missing only two more ticks. According to this record, it had now been five months and twenty-eight days since I had received my diagnosis. This would allot me two more days of life. Perhaps out of some ancient superstition I was not ready to scoff at this prospect. However, unless lightning were to strike me or a lioness managed to make a meal of my now much tougher muscles, I perceived no indication of impending death. On the contrary, I was feeling better, stronger, and more positive with each passing day. I would celebrate, I decided—in two days.

My greatly improved physical condition was due largely to my long walks around the neighborhood, the weeding and planting in my small garden, and other physical chores.

Each day I had to walk far to pick fresh fruit or dig up a tuber, to examine the various traps I managed to construct for catching an impressive assortment of small animals, and to follow my greatest passion: fishing.

I remembered my first days here, when my entire body ached each morning as a result of even a short hike. But with time my walks got longer until I was able to sustain many miles of travel without any discomfort.

X visited me again on the first day of my seventh month here.

"You have survived your death sentence," he said with an uplifting tone of voice. "Congratulations are in order."

"By one day so far," I said.

"I am sure there will be many more. You have made tremendous progress already—your diet, your physical activity."

I had to agree with his assessment. I even began to enjoy all of it.

"I often wonder why people back home lead such sedentary lifestyles," I said. "It seems so unnatural and so self-sabotaging. Just think, no animals out here develop any chronic diseases. They die of old age or as the victims of their natural predators. They never develop any habits that would be harmful to their existence and survival. There are no sedentary cheetahs or obese antelopes. Nature's laws of survival would not tolerate such deviations from the norm."

"You have become very observant," X agreed. "In fact, most species maintain delicate balances within their habitats by keeping each other in check. Consider an area where rabbits and foxes coexist. An unexpected overabundance of rabbits does not cause the fox population to become lazy and obese. On the contrary, they rapidly multiply, dramatically reduce the rabbit population, and so their next generation must again work very hard just to survive. These predator-prey cycles govern all life on our planet."

"So how can you explain that humans have been able to escape from these basic laws of nature?" I asked.

"As with food, it is again largely due to our intelligence. Through the ages, we have been able to change our environment to the point where physical activity is hardly a necessity. Until some 10,000 years ago, we had lived as hunters and gatherers, depending on nature and simple weapons for our survival. This required a lot of demanding physical activity. The development of agriculture made food supply more predictable but producing it still required a lot of hard physical labor. Next, the Industrial Revolution caused a major shift from the farms to factories and produced machines to make the production of food more efficient. Yet the majority of the population was still required to perform much physical work. Only the last few decades—the age of computers and robots—made it possible for most people to live their entire lives without doing any serious physical work. Unfortunately, evolution is too slow to keep up with this explosive development. The human body has not changed in any significant way since the times of the early hunters and gatherers and it is poorly adapted to the environment most people live in."

"Yeah, that all makes a lot of sense. But we can't wind the clock back thousands of years. What's the solution?"

"Have you ever subscribed to a gym membership?" X asked.

I nodded sheepishly.

"I gather it has not lasted very long," X guessed correctly. "Do you know why?"

I did but wanted to hear his explanation.

"It's very simple—you didn't enjoy it. "And as long as you think of exercise as an unpleasant necessity, you can always conjure up some excuse to skip it—too much work, need to spend time with the kids, feeling depressed."

"That's all accurate," I said "but I am not hearing what the alternative is."

"We all are fighting a powerful evolutionary instinct—not to waste energy. This instinct made a lot of sense when nutrition was scarce but in an environment of unlimited calories it is working against us. The only hope to fight this instinct is to find a physical activity that we would find rewarding and so we would be willing to perform voluntarily and regularly. Back home, you could have possibly found something you would enjoy—if not the gym then perhaps some hiking, or swimming, or biking—who knows. But there was no time to let you find out on your own. You had to act, rapidly and unequivocally, and that's why you are here."

"That certainly worked for me. I look forward to each and every day. But let's say I do actually return back home someday. Wouldn't I succumb to the same old temptations of laziness and indolence?" I asked.

"I doubt it." X said. "Once you have discovered the pleasure of physical activities, you will want to maintain them for as long as you live."

I tried to remember when was the last time I did something physically demanding back home. I did play some sports in high school, even college, mostly a few rounds of tennis or the occasional swim. When was the last time I did a serious hike? I had only fuzzy memories of walks in the local mountains with my parents, none of which had left any lasting impressions.

After college, I felt the need to spend every waking hour on building my career. Physical activity was not on my mind until I noticed my belly fat accumulate too prodigiously. But at that time I had already been plagued by too many aches and pains, things I automatically attributed to my middle age: an aching lower back, pain in my right knee when walking up the stairs, and frequent headaches. All of these were most convenient excuses for not running, hiking, biking, or even taking a walk on the beach.

Now, after just a few months in my new environment, I could see clearly that it was precisely the lack of physical activity that let my body deteriorate to the point of needing frequent medical intervention. But I also discovered an invaluable truth: it was not too late for me to reverse the downward spiral of my earlier life. I was sure my body was still capable of repairing the damage of years of neglect.

***

TOne morning I ventured unusually far from my hut. I kept climbing a gradually rising incline. Each time I thought I had reached the edge, another range opened up just above it. By the time I reached the summit, the sun had already begun its rapid descent toward the distant horizon. Despite the large distance, I could still make out my hut far in the distance. I was trying to judge how far I had to walk to get back and just then I noticed something unusual in front of the hut's door. There was some motion. I strained my eyes against the sun's orange glare. Perhaps it was just my imagination, an optical illusion created by the setting sun. But no, there it was again. Something was definitely moving in front of the door. Some animal looking for scraps of food, I reasoned.

I resumed my brisk walk and as I got closer, I recognized a shape—a human shape—a yellow skirt, a colorful blouse. I was shocked. There was a girl, a small girl standing in front of my hut! I broke into a trot. After a few minutes I saw that she was watching me. I slowed down, not wanting to frighten her, but she remained there, motionless. She was leaning against the door, with her hands behind her back, completely still, but her eyes were following my approach expectantly, as if she already knew me. She seemed very young, perhaps seven or eight years of age, if I had to guess.

I stopped a few steps in front of her and looked around. There was no one else. How in the world did she get here alone? And why?

"Hello, sweetie," I said tentatively, looking into her large dark eyes. Her long eye lashes sank as she looked down at the ground in front of her small bare feet. Would she even understand English? I took another step forward and let myself down on one knee in front of her.

"Selami?" I said, trying one of the few words I picked up from X. At this, her eyes shot upward and she looked directly into my eyes.

"Selami," she said almost cheerfully.

"Ok, Selami," I repeated and gently touched her cheek with the back of my fingers. It felt like touching golden velvet. She had a delicate round face with beautifully carved puffy lips.

I stood up and, looking around one more time to assure myself that she was indeed alone, I tried to conjure some explanation for this most unexpected visit. Could she be simply lost? It was hard to imagine a child this young having walked for miles through the wilderness, but children have been known to accomplish remarkable feats when challenged. But why? And more importantly, what should I do now?

I rose and pointed to the path leading from the distant hills. "Have you come from there?"

She looked puzzled but as I repeatedly pointed at her and at the distant horizon, she made the connection and a glimmer of understanding appeared on her lips. She nodded. "Mbala dubu," she added.

"Bala dubu?" I repeated and she nodded. "What in the world does that mean," I said, more to myself then to her. "Bala dubu, heh? Ok. I have no idea if this is a place, or your name, or the reason why you are here, but at least we are talking, right?" She looked at me quizzically but a hint of a smile seemed to have formed around her mouth.

"Ok, baby." I let myself down on my knee again, facing her squarely. "My name is Richard, ok?" Then, pointing repeatedly at my chest, I repeated. "Richard. Richard." She studied me intently but I indicated that I wanted her to repeat my words. "Richard." I said again, stabbing my chest with my index finger.

Tentatively, she obeyed. "Richah."

"Excellent, girl, excellent," I exclaimed and made her repeat my name again.

"Richah, Richah," she chanted, now more confidently.

"That's it. Richard. And now you, princess. What is your name?" I pointed at her chest and repeated my question. "Your name?"

"Nyala." She smiled as she pronounced her name with obvious pride.

"How pretty," I exclaimed excited at my success. "Nyala. Hmm, I really like the sound of it. We could be friends, you know. If you could only explain to me who you are and what you are doing here, in the middle of nowhere, all alone."

As no explanation was forthcoming, I opened the door to my hut.

"Enter my palace, mysterious little princes," I said and gestured to make my invitation understandable. Nyala took a few steps forward and stopped in the middle of the room, taking in the new surroundings. I took her by the hand and led her to the mat in the corner of the room that served as my bed and motioned for her to sit down. She sat with her legs crossed and her back straight as an arrow, as if attempting a yoga exercise.

"Hungry?" I inquired mostly rhetorically. "Of course you are hungry. You must have walked a few miles to get here. Unless of course you have been dropped off by aliens, which I seriously doubt. So, here we go…"

I broke off a piece of cassava cake, which I had learned to make in a long trial-and-error process, and offered it to Nyala, along with a banana. She took both politely but immediately tore into both, alternating her bites between the patty and fruit.

"Good girl." I poured her a cup of goat milk, which she drank with relish in long noisy gulps.

I wiped the white mustache from her lips with the back of my hand.

"So, what do you want to do now, princess?" I was beginning to enjoy my monologues with this mysterious creature. Perhaps she was a fairy and this was just a test for me. Who knows, if I treated her well, she might have granted me a wish, or even three.

I went back to the cupboard to prepare some supper for myself. I sliced off another piece of the cassava cake and added some vegetables I had just finished harvesting from my garden. I put everything on a plate, ready to sit down and continue my one-sided conversation with my new guest. But when I turned around to face her, she was no longer sitting. She was lying on her side, with her knees pulled up to her chest and her hands tucked away between her knees. Poor thing, I thought as I watched her little body rise and fall gently with each breath. She must have been totally exhausted to just keel over and fall asleep within seconds. What a day—for both of us.

***

When I woke up, expecting X's familiar face next to me, I was surprised to be looking at Nyala. She was kneeling next to my bed, watching me sleep. This was no dream.

"Good morning, my princess," I said and stretched out my arm to stroke her cheek.

She smiled in return, but there was a hint of anxiety in her expression.

I rose to a half-sitting position to see her better.

"What's wrong, baby?"

She said nothing, just kept looking at me intently.

"What is it?" I repeated more urgently and made gestures to let her know that I wanted to know if anything was the matter. She pointed to the door.

"You want to go out?" I said and mimicked walking with my two fingers on the pillow.

She nodded emphatically.

I got up, put on my shirt and pants, and pointed toward the table. "Breakfast?"

She shook he head and pointed to the door again.

"What's the hurry?" I said, more to myself then to her, but she had already taken my hand to make me follow her.

She started to walk in a direction away from the stream.

"Where are you taking me?" I asked, pointing toward the horizon and making an inquiring gesture.

"Dini," she said and pointed forward.

"Dini?" I repeated. "What in the world is that?"

But she kept walking, now more hastily than before. We walked for a long time, the sun was now high in the sky and I regretted not having taken my hat. I would pay for this with a nasty sunburn. We crossed a little stream I didn't even know about. We drank from the clear water but Nyala granted us only a few minutes' rest.

About an hour later, she slowed down, as if trying to recognize something. The surrounding countryside was arid with occasional islands of green vegetation. I had visited this place once or twice before but remembered nothing special about it.

Suddenly she veered from the path and began to run toward a large cluster of tall trees. I tried to follow but she was too agile for me. A moment later I saw her disappear in the dense bushes of the little oasis.

"Nyala," I called out when I reached the point where she dove in.

There was no reply. Cautiously I pushed away the thorny branches to be able to advance. Then I spotted the yellow dress. She was kneeling on the ground, examining something.

"Nyala," I said reproachfully. "What's all this—?" Before I could complete my reprimand, I recognized that she was bent over a human body. I came closer and squatted next to her to see who it was.

"Dini," she said again. There were tears in her eyes.

On the ground before us, bedded on a layer of leaves and shielded from the sun by the thick canopy above, was an old woman, her eyes half closed. She was breathing laboriously.

There was no point in trying to understand who this was. Dini. A relative perhaps, or a friend. Nyala must have left her here yesterday before she came to my hut.

I reached out and placed my palm on the old woman's furrowed forehead. She was burning with fever. I dribbled some water into her mouth from my bottle. She swallowed eagerly. Nyala looked at me with deep brown eyes as if I was the Savior himself.

"We need to take her home," I said. She was a small person but still, the hut was hours away. I thought of improvising some sort of a stretcher but when I looked at Nyala's tiny body, I rejected the idea. Some sort of a travois to drag behind me? In the hurried departure I didn't even think of bringing my knife.

In the end I just picked up Dini, and with Nyala's help, hoisted her on my back. She was lighter than I expected. I put my arms under her stick-like thighs, locked my hands in front of my stomach, and started to walk back.

Dini was able to hold on with her arms and I felt her hot breath as she leaned her chin on my shoulder.

I walked slowly, knowing that I had to stretch my remaining strength to make it home. I could not look back but was aware of Nyala's steps following close behind me.

I had to take a break every half hour. We all drank some water and I lay flat on the ground, trying to relax my cramped muscles. I watched the sun patiently making its way toward the horizon and with every passing hour my doubts that we could make it before sunset increased.

When the colors finally faded from the landscape, I was sure. We had to sleep out in the open. Before complete darkness swallowed us, I chose an island of trees, similar to where we found Dini. We gathered some dry leaves to soften the ground and lay down to sleep, Nyala wedged between me and Dini, who now seemed to be in a state of semi-consciousness.

I stroked Nyala's smooth hair. She was breathing quietly and the rhythmic motion of her tiny body pressing tightly against me soon put me to sleep as well.

When I opened my eyes, the first light was already breaking through the dense foliage overhead. Nyala was seated on the ground with her back toward me. I reached out and let my palm run gently up and down her spine.

"Good morning, princess," I said. "You're up early."

She didn't stir. I got up and sat beside her, putting my arm around her tiny shoulders. She rubbed her eyes with the palms of her hands.

"What's wrong, baby?"

I looked at Dini. She was lying in front of us, her eyes closed. I looked back at Nyala. Her profile was partially hidden by a lock of long hair. She seemed to be crying noiselessly. Then it began to dawn on me. Dini's chest was no longer moving. I touched her hand—it was cold.

We both remained seated at Dini's side for a long time.

"Poor child," I only managed to whisper. "Why?"

I didn't know what to do. Carrying a lifeless body, no matter how light, was beyond my physical strength. We would have to bury her here. But how?

I took Nyala into my arms and stroked her hair consolingly. She was quiet now, stoically composed. Using gestures, I tried to make her understand what I had to do. She agreed. We decided to leave Dini in the place where she passed away. We spent several hours gathering rocks in the area. We covered the body with a layer of dry leaves, on top of which we piled the rocks to form a protective tomb. I broke off two straight branches and laid them on top in the form of a cross. Nyala looked at me quizzically. I had no way of explaining my action, so I just pointed both palms upward toward the sky. She nodded.

Before leaving, we both kneeled at the foot of the grave and sunk into private thoughts.

X seemed sad that night as well.

"Why do things have to be so difficult sometimes," I asked, not really expecting an answer.

"Things usually happen for a reason," X said, "and every dark moment is followed by a light one."

I sighed. Words of wisdom, but they sounded hollow.

X read my thoughts as he continued.

"The light moment for you is Nyala. She must now become the center of your life."

"She is wonderful." I nodded.

"And she is totally alone in this world. There is no one to help her survive but you. You are her world."

"Don't worry," I said. "I will try my best."

"No. Your best is not enough. A great burden has been placed upon you. If you die, she will die too. Do you grasp the enormity of this responsibility? Now it's not just you and your health. Now there is another helpless human being totally dependent on your well-bring. Now you are simply not allowed to die."

How old was Nyala? I failed to communicate my question to her using signs, perhaps she didn't even know. I would place her somewhere within the first few grades of elementary education but she was very mature for whatever age she might be.

The morning after our return from the funeral, she was already outside when I woke up. I stepped out to check what she was up to. I found her kneeling at the side of the goat, which she had tied to the fence. She was milking her. The bowl under the udder was already half full and each new squeeze of her little hand added another squirt.

"Where have you learned to do that," I asked.

She looked up smiling sweetly but continued the task. When the bowl was almost full, she stood up and held it up to my face.

"Should I drink this?" I asked.

She shook her head and just carried the bowl back to the hut where she covered it with a cloth. It would be spoiled quickly in the heat, I was sure, but I didn't want to dampen her enthusiasm.

In the evening, Nyala surprised me again with her astuteness. As I had predicted, the milk had already turned sour. Unsightly whitish lumps were now floating in a cloudy whey. Instead of throwing it away, as I was about to do, she spread the cloth over another bowl and strained the sour milk. She wrapped the while lumps into the cloth and twisted it to wring out as much of the liquid as possible. She then hung the bundle on a string.

I had only a vague idea of how cheese was made but this seemed like the first step. Nyala confirmed my guess the next morning when she unwrapped the bundle. Most of the liquid had now dripped out. What remained was a generous portion of fresh cheese. She mixed it with the chopped leaves of some plant she had picked up outside and let me taste it.

It was delicious and inspiring.

"Let me show you what we eat at Thanksgiving," I told her, knowing full well that she had no idea what I was talking about.

I strode out to the garden and carefully pulled four large yams out of the ground. I gathered some dry leaves and branches and made a fire. When the flamed died down, I placed the yams on the hot ambers, turning them with a stick once in a while to bake them evenly. An hour later, we sat down in the grass, cut open the now soft tubers, and covered their orange insides with Nyala's cheese. It was the most rewarding Thanksgiving feast of my life.

I noticed with boundless satisfaction that this was the very first time in my life when Thanksgiving was not an empty and mostly bothersome obligation to either visit or to host some distant relatives, to eat and drink to the point of numb stupor, and to swear that next year would be different. Here for the first time in my life I experienced the true meaning of giving thanks for something significant. There was no pressure and no pretense to feel anything, just a warm glow that slowly permeated my entire body in a wave of unrestrained bliss. I was thankful for being here, for having Nyala at my side, for being alive.

***

Today was a very special day for me. When I updated my wall calendar, as I did every evening before going to sleep, I completed the last mark of the sixth row. I have now been here for six entire months. There was no need to be superstitious any longer—I had survived the six months allotted to me by Dr. Green's prognosis.

I put down the piece of charcoal I used to make the last mark and lay on my mat. Nyala was already sleep, I heard her relaxed breathing in the darkness.

How could our medicine be so wrong? How did they even dare to make a prediction about life and death?

I recalled the story of the little girl, walking on the beach strewn with thousands of stranded sand dollar shells. She kept picking them up and throwing them back into the sea.

"Why do you do that?" asked her mother.

"I am saving them," said the girl.

"But there are way too many. You can't make a difference," objected her mother.

"But I can make a difference to this one," said the girl as she picked up another sand dollar and threw it back into safety.

Tonight I felt like one of the lucky sand dollars that got another chance.

Recently, I began to feel very much in peace with myself. I contributed that in part to my undisturbed and most restful sleep each night. Not having any artificial light, my daily rhythm was dictated largely by the sun. At times I let a small fire burn for a while after sunset, and I watched the flames slowly quiet down, until only the red embers remained to bathe the hut in a warm glow. But most of the evenings I just sat outside the hut and watched the sky gradually lose its brightness, the pale blue hues transforming into orange and red in the west and dark blue in the east. When all the blue turned gray and eventually black, with only billions of bright pinholes of distant stars illuminating the landscape, I went inside and drifted into sleep. I had watched this transformation hundreds of times but each time it was a magically tranquilizing event, something I had never experience in my life at home. Even far away from city lights, during camping, the darkness was always disturbed by flashlights, phone screens, and other annoying electronics.

Even more magical was the moment of sunrise, which I had never really appreciated before—the moment when the first pink rays of the sun breach the horizon and nature begins to stir in myriads of animal and insect sounds.

I began to realize how absurdly unnatural my sleeping habits were back home. I went to bed late, usually after working at the computer well past midnight. Then I woke up to the unrelenting beeping of the alarm clock. I used to hate the mornings with a vengeance. Every morning I dragged myself out of bed depressed and angry at the world. There was no rest and nothing to look forward to other than more work. I also frequently woke up in the middle of the night and realized with annoyance that my brain was still processing some of the problems I had left unfinished the preceding day. Sleep was not a time of rest, but a form of torture.

I recounted my observations to X and he only nodded in sympathy.

"Sleep is greatly undervalued in your society," he said. "People boast about how little sleep they need, presumably to show how strong and productive they are. But they are just fooling themselves."

"I certainly appreciate my restful sleep," I said, "but, honestly, back home I could not have afforded to go to bed with the sunset and wake up on my own, just whenever my body would feel like it."

"But you could afford to get sick, end up here, and be forced to sleep the way your body was designed to?"

He was right, of course. Sleep was not very high on my list of priorities and a convenient excuse for staying up late was always at hand. But why would it be such a big deal?

"Are you suggesting that I got cancer because of a lack of sleep?" I asked.

"No," he said patiently, "but it most likely contributed to it."

"How could that be?" I said, thinking that X was taking mostly in hyperbole.

"There are several types of sleep—I assume you are familiar with that?"

"Well, I know there is REM sleep during which your eyes show some strange rapid movements, I think. What else?"

"Yes, REM sleep is when you dream. Then there is light sleep and deep sleep," he elaborated.

"Ok, and?"

"It's the deep sleep that's the most important. This is a somewhat mysterious phase during which the brain produces high-amplitude, low-frequency delta waves. You do know about brain waves, don't you?"

"I know that the EEG measures brain waves but that's about the extent of my knowledge of neurology," I said.

"That will do," X continued. "What matters is that during deep sleep the growth hormone is released into your bloodstream and that, my friend, promotes cell repair in your body. So enough deep sleep is crucial for restoring you both physically and mentally."

"So lack of proper sleep made me feel miserable every morning back home? That would certainly explain why I have not been experiencing any blues lately."

"I am sure that's a big part of it, plus the fact that your worries out here do not overwhelm you."

"And you really think that lack of deep sleep also contributed to my disease?"

"I am convinced of that," X said. "Lack of deep sleep is linked to many chronic problems—heart disease, high blood pressure, obesity, diabetes, Alzheimer's. If your hormone balances get out of whack, anything can go wrong. In your case, deep sleep probably saved you by boosting your immune system."

"I certainly appreciate my new-found well-being but I'm worried about the future. How will I sustain this should I ever go back home?"

"You will," X assured me with a pat on my back. "Stop working well before you go to bed to let your brain wind down. Don't look at your cellphone or tablet or any screen during the night or in the late evening—those screens emit a lot of light frequencies that interfere with your circadian rhythm, your internal bio-clocks, which in turn messes up your hormone levels—melatonin and such."

"Anything else?"

"Just follow your body's demands and your mind's common sense. They know best what they need and what's ultimately good for your heath."

***

As the days passed, I got used to my new diet of fruits and vegetables, nuts, sweet potatoes, the occasional egg, and a steady supply of fish. I felt light inside and out. Flashbacks of fat burgers with fries and buckets of milkshakes that used to torture me during my first weeks here have all faded away. They turned into strange comic strips I could only laugh about. But there was one thing I still missed: good bread. Visions of dark crusty breads, crispy baguettes, or yellow cornbread kept pursuing me every night.

I decided to try my luck at baking. Unfortunately, the only grains I had available were sorghum and corn. The corn was now well past ripe, some of the ears were becoming hard and dry. I picked a few of the most mature ones and using my knife, stripped off the kernels into a bowl. I also tossed in a handful of sorghum.

I walked out and selected a large flat rock onto which I carefully emptied a portion of the kernels. With a round stone I began to grind them down. I was hoping for some kind of flower but the kernels still contained much moisture and turned into a firm sticky mush. I scooped it out back into the bowl, added some water and two eggs, and kneaded everything into a yellowy dough.

All this time, Nyala was squatting next to me, observing my activity with great curiosity.

"Baby," I said, "I don't really know what I am doing here. A science experiment, I suppose."

I kept turning the dough around in the bowl, uncertain of what to do next.

"We don't have an oven," I said, looking at Nyala. "What now?"

She seemed to grasp my dilemma and pointed to the fireplace in the hut.

"I know," I said, "we do have fire but how do we bake bread on an open fire?"

The fireplace only had a grill, which was good enough for roasting sweet potatoes or fish, but my dough was not firm enough to form a loaf. She didn't understand and so I mimed slapping the dough on the grill. She laughed and ran off. She broke off a huge leaf from a nearby plant and spread it out flat on the ground. She took the bowl from my hands, dumped its contents onto the center of the leaf, and skillfully folded its sides into an envelope. She lifted the bundle carefully onto the grill and placed a little stone on top of it to prevent the leaf from unfolding. She looked at me expectantly.

"Clever girl," I said with genuine admiration. "Let the baking begin."

I lit a low fire under the leaf and we let it bake until the leaf started to turn black. When the fire died down, I carefully peeled back the blackened sides of the leaf, exposing a brownish yellow loaf of what I declared our sorghum-corn experiment. I almost burned my fingers as I tried to break off a piece to taste it. It had a hard crust on the outside but the inside was still undercooked and far from appetizing. I offered a piece to Nyala who sniffed it suspiciously.

"I don't think this would sell well at a Paris boulangerie," I said as I chewed on our creation. "How do you like it?"

Nyala nodded politely.

"Great. I suggest we take the rest of the day off."

***

Nyala must have slipped out early in the morning because I had not heard her get up. This was nothing unusual, she often got up long before me and went out in search of fruits or other edibles. When she returned late in the afternoon, she was carrying a large bag in front of her.

"What have you got there?" I asked with undisguised

curiosity.

"Bread," she said. She had picked up many words from my constant monologues and tried to apply them to improve our communication.

"Bread?" I said with amusement, assuming she must have misunderstood the word.

She opened the bag to show me its contents. It was filled with tiny round kernels, something I had only seen in pet shops sold as food for hamsters or birds.

"Is that millet?" I asked.

"This is zinijero," Nyala said.

"Hmm, if you say so." I picked up a few kernels and popped them into my mouth. They were hard as buck shot and Nyala laughed as I spit them out.

She picked up the bag and carried it out to the large flat rock we used yesterday to mash our corn. She put a handful into a shallow depression, picked up a round stone, and started to grind them down. A minute later the depression was filled with a coarse yellowy flower.

Encouraged by the result, I picked up another stone and imitated her effort using a different spot. Less than half an hour later, we had a small bag of flower, ready to be made into a dough. Nyala mixed it using only water and a handful of some other tiny poppy-like seeds she had also gathered during her morning walk. I only watched with fascination as she skillfully formed the firm dough into several patties the size of pita bread.

I had no idea how she intended to bake them but she exuded confidence. She started a fire and asked me to help her carry a large flat rock, which we placed on top of the low-burning wood. When the fire died down, she slapped one of the flat breads onto the hot stone. It sizzled momentarily and small bubbles started to rise to its surface. When the edges turned brown and began to lift from the hot surface, she slipped a forked branch under it and turned it over. A minute later, she lifted it with the branch and held it up to let it cool down. She broke it in half and offered one to me.

"This is still far from a crusty rye bread but it's delicious," I said with my mouth still full. I took her face into my hands, pulled her toward me, and gave her a kiss on the forehead.

"You are my bread fairy," I said as she put her arms around me in a tight embrace. It was the sweetest moment of my life.

***

There was so much happening in my new life now that I hadn't noticed X's prolonged absence. I was pleasantly surprised to see him again at my bedside.

"I noticed you have been rather busy lately," he said "so I didn't want to intrude."

"Oh, don't be silly. You are always more than welcome in my home," I countered. "Your insights have been invaluable to my survival so I am more than curious to hear what you have for me this time?"

X smiled gently.

"I must admit that you have surpassed even my most optimistic expectations," he said. "Your excellent diet, your increased physical activity, your mental state, and your attachment to the child, all those have turned your life around. You will make it, I am sure of it."

"I agree with you one hundred percent. But at times I still feel anxious, unable to sleep. I worry about what will come next."

"Do you know the real meaning of stress?" X asked.

I thought about if for a moment.

"Back home," I said, "it was simply the pressures of daily life—unfinished work piling up, deadlines, family demands, bills to pay—things like that."

"But that's not stress," X replied. "All these negative pressures and demands are the stressors—something that interferes with your body's equilibrium. Stress is the body's reaction to the stressors."

That seemed like a minor semantic point but I let X continue.

"Do you remember your encounter with the lioness?" He asked.

"Do I! I was scared shitless," I admitted.

"You recall your heart pounding uncontrollably, your muscles tensing, and cold sweat bathing your skin—that was the stress response, automatic and completely beyond your control."

"Yes, the old fight-or-flight response. But isn't that totally different from say, trying to meet a deadline at work?" I said.

"Not really. When you get an unexpected call from your boss to come to his office right away, what's your immediate unconscious reaction—increased heartbeat, clammy palms, dry mouth, a slight panic attack—perhaps not as dramatic as during your lioness encounter but in essence the same. Later you calm down and everything seems back to normal."

"Right. So what's the problem? The fight-or-flight response is just a very natural defense mechanism that prepares a person, or any animal for that matter, to deal with an impending danger. It mobilizes the body's resources for a physical fight or to run away. Am I right?"

"Absolutely," X assented.

"So if this is a perfectly normal and natural reaction, my body should know how to get back to normal once the danger passes. Why would this be damaging to my body?"

"Do you know how the brain accomplishes the fight-or-flight response?"

I had some vague ideas but since I didn't respond, X continued.

"It's hormones. Your brain controls your body by releasing a host of different hormones into your bloodstream."

"Like adrenaline?" I asked.

"That and many others. The problem is that while releasing them takes seconds, getting them back to normal levels takes hours, even days, especially if the perceived danger just passes and no physical action—no fight and no flight—actually takes place."

"Is it the frequency of the stressful events that's the problem?"

"That and the intensity, of course. Let's say you hear a

burglar in your house. That can be extremely frightening, but a one-time occurrence will not cause any damage to your body's biochemistry. But imagine having to live with the fear of burglary on a daily basis."

"You would get used to it, I suppose."

"You may think so but your body doesn't. It needs time to recover from a stress response. It must clear all the stress-related hormones form the blood stream and permit all the biochemical processes involved in the response to return to a normal steady state. When a stress trigger repeats too frequently, or when a collection of different triggers accumulates within a short time interval, or when the stress situation is very long, the brain doesn't have a chance to shut down the stress response. Consequently, the body is constantly flooded with stress hormones and remains in a permanent state of high alert, unnatural nervousness, and anxiety. This is chronic stress."

"And this is related to cancer?"

X shrugged noncommittally.

"Possibly. Nobody knows for certain and most chronic diseases are just too complex to be pinned down to one single cause. But just think of the mess you are making in your body when you keep stressing it. It keeps releasing the hormone vasopressin, which, as its name suggests, influences blood pressure and heart rate. So think heart disease. It also releases thyroxin, which influences the body's metabolism, increases mental alertness, anxiety, irritability, and disturbs sleep. It releases cortisol, which increases fats in the blood and impacts your immune system. Do I need to go on?"

This explanation was most enlightening but opened even more new questions. Was I still under too much stress out here, worried about my daily survival, Nyala's well-being, my cancer situation, my future? Before I could ask any more, X had already vanished; I would have to wait until the next time we met.

***

During my extended walks I learned to listen more

attentively to the cacophony of sounds surrounding me. I began to differentiate between the various bird, insect, and frog sounds, many of which I could link to particular times of day or night. On many occasions I tried to imitate some of them, with varying success. There was one particular bird with a high-pitched squeak, which I was able to imitate by whistling closely enough to elicit a response. It felt good to be able to finally communicate with another living being, even if it was only a small elusive bird that rarely showed its yellow and green plumage.

I realized how much I missed music. Real music, with a rhythm and a melody. I had never learned to play any musical instrument well. As a child I was forced to take a few keyboard lessons but the seeming uselessness of this task stifled my progress only too quickly. In college I tried my luck with a guitar, mostly because of a girl who adored rock stars, but I would be hard-pressed to strike even a simple e-major chord now.

Still, I needed music in my life and I began to think about the possibility of making some musical instrument. Given my knowledge and the very limited tools at my disposal, a string instrument was clearly out of my league. Perhaps some wind instrument, a simple flute. As children, we learned how to make whistles from soft willow branches by loosening the bark until the wooden core could be pulled out, thus creating a hollow tube. Then by cutting holes into the bark and replacing portions of the core, the tube could be fashioned into a whistle. But even the most skilled among us couldn't get more than a few shrill notes out of these creations.

I would have to resort to percussion. Just about anything could make a sound when struck the right way and so I went on a search for suitable material. It would have to be hollow and preferably light-weight. I had a large gourd that I used occasionally to store water. I made a couple of small holes along its open edge so I could hang it from a branch. I hit it with a stick and it responded with a surprisingly full-bodied sound. I tried a few more taps, striking it in different places, and was pleased with the outcome of my endeavor.

Buoyed by initial success, I decided to make a pair of larger drums, aiming for something resembling the congas I had always admired in Caribbean music. It took me a long time and much banging on tree trunks during my daily walks through the forest before I found one whose trunk seemed hollow and that wasn't too large for me to handle. It seemed mostly dead, with just a few green leaves at its very top. The trunk felt very dry to the touch and light when I tapped it. With a few careful hits of my machete I cut off the top and peered inside. It was indeed completely hollow. I made another cut further below, which resulted in a tube some three feet in height and almost a foot in diameter—a perfect start for a conga drum.

I carefully chipped at the rim for a while, making it as even as I could manage with my primitive tools, and carried my creation back to the hut. There I cut out a circular piece of hide large enough to cover the opening of the wooden trunk. I cut small holes, about one inch apart along the perimeter of the hide and used long strings, cut from the same hide, to spread the skin over the open top of the trunk. This proved to be the most frustrating part of the project, as each string had to be fed under the bottom of the trunk and tied progressively tighter at each step to make sure the skin was spread not only very tightly but evenly along the entire perimeter of the opening.

Despite my best effort, I was not able to achieve the necessary tension to create a crisp sound when striking the skin with my palms or even with an improvised mallet. Disappointed, I put my creation outside, determined to work on it again the next day.

A stroke of luck helped me to solve the problem. A heavy rain soaked everything outside, including my new conga drum. The skin became very soft, drooping in the middle under the weight of the puddle of water that had gathered there overnight. I wiped it away and retightened the now limp strings. After letting it dry out in the sun for a few hours I tried to tap it again. The skin now felt as tight as a sheet of polished metal and a few excited taps with my fingers gave off a volley of sharp full-bodied sounds that made a nearby flock of birds explode in a panicked flight.

Little Nyala broke out into a spontaneous dance when I demonstrated my creation with utmost pride. I had not felt so much unrestrained happiness since the days of my childhood. In my previous life, music was just an omnipresent commodity, a consumer good, accessible in all forms any time of day or night, yet I never fully appreciated it. Here I felt it was a form of communication older than even spoken language. As I immersed myself into more and more complicated rhythms, all my worries began to fade and my mind started to dissolve into a state of all-encompassing tranquility.

That night, as I lay in my cot relaxed after my musical experience, I recalled my conversation with X about stress. If stress is such an important mechanism that protects us and all living beings from danger, why did people turn it into something so harmful?

was happy to provide some insights into this puzzle. "Because we are too intelligent," he said simply.

This made little sense so I asked him to elaborate.

"Animals respond to threats that are real. Only people are capable of imagining threats that may never happen or are even physically impossible. A dog will have a stress reaction when faced with a snake and so will you. But only you can visualize a snake encounter and have the same stress reaction as if it was real. You can think of the consequences of this encounter, the pain or death resulting from a bite, the tragic consequences for your family. You can even imagine a snake with unrealistic properties and behaviors. There is no limit to human imagination. Real threats are a much smaller problem than threats fabricated by our intelligent minds."

"So I can have a stress reaction by just thinking about something terrible?"

"Absolutely. But there is more. Think about how we deal with stress. Animals follow their instincts. If they perceive something as dangerous or uncomfortable, they run away or try to fight it off to the best of their abilities. But we can't always do that and so we must suppress our instincts. When faced with an intimidating boss, you do not simply run away. You can foresee the potential consequences and this stops you from doing what your body is prepared to do—fight or flight. Instead, you force yourself to overcome the aversion and suppress any immediate desire to relieve the stress."

"Luckily I don't have a boss here," I said with great satisfaction, "and no hateful flare-ups to suppress."

"Exactly. And you also have no deadlines, no financial worries, no pollution or traffic noise, no enemies to deal with—"

"You don't need to continue," I interrupted. I glanced through the window at the sky sparkling with stars and listened to the noise of the night. "I know where I am. But I still feel stressed at times, about finding enough to eat, getting injured, things like that."

"Of course you do and that's perfectly normal. This is a low level of stress, designed to help your body adapt to the ever-changing world around you. Everyone experiences some level of stress every day, be it the crossing of a busy intersection or witnessing a child scrape his knee. As long as this stress level is low, your body can easily handle it and, if the same stressor repeats frequently, the brain gradually adapts to it so you no longer perceive it with the same intensity. You become desensitized. This gradual adaptation permits you to overcome fears and with time permits you to act in ways you could have never imagined possible.

"This low level of stress, which serves as an adaptation and motivational force, is sometimes called the good stress. The boundary between good stress and bad, however, is not sharp. As the intensity or frequency of stressors increases, the stress level continues to rise. At some point it ceases to be a positive driving force and turns into a negative one, which gets in the way of your progress."

"I had never thought of stress as something positive—a

protective or adaptive mechanism," I admitted.

"But you must be very careful to keep it within an optimal range—a level that the body can manage without harm."

"How would I know if I am still within that healthy range?"

X took a deep breath before plunging into an extensive elaboration.

"Stress is largely a matter of perception," he began. "What I mean is, your body's reaction to a given stressor is very subjective and varies widely from person to person. Getting lost in the wilderness and having to spend the night alone could be a terrifying ordeal for an urbanite who has never left the comforts of civilization. But the same situation could be just an interesting diversion for an experienced survivalist who has the necessary level of knowledge, skills, and experience to make it back to safety."

"So what I'm hearing you say is that stress depends on how well I can deal with a given unexpected situation?"

"Exactly. Imagine two curves on a graph, one representing the level of your stressors and the other your resources to handle the demands. When I say resources I don't mean time or money, but rather thigs that are mostly intangible—your knowledge, skills, and experiences accumulated throughout your lifetime. Both curves will fluctuate up or down through the course of your lifetime and both have a tendency to rise gradually as new knowledge, skills, and material wealth are acquired. But the level of your stress does not depend on how high or low either curve is. Rather, it depends on the distance between the two. In an ideal situation, the stress curve will be only slightly above the resource curve and this moderate stress will serve you as a motivating factor. But when the stress curve suddenly shoots up or continues rising faster than your resources, you are in trouble. This is chronic stress and it will make you sick in more ways than you can imagine."

"This all makes a lot of sense but given the great harm that stress can cause, I can only wonder why people are willing to accept so much of it in their lives."

"That's a complicated question with roots in psychology,

economics, and sometimes just pure ignorance. Many people, especially men, feel they are strong enough to take all the pressures of life by essentially ignoring them and might even feel like weaklings and cowards if they tried to seek help. They would scoff at the suggestion of engaging in any type of stress reduction activities. Another reason is that effective stress management requires effort and time, which most people are unwilling to invest. Paradoxically, it is typically the lack of time itself that causes much of the stress. The common response 'I am simply too stressed to engage in any stress reduction' captures the dilemma. Finally, stress can become an addiction in itself. Just like a person may become addicted to chocolate, drugs, gambling, or work, it is also possible to become addicted to stress itself and to actively seek out stressful situations as a personal challenge."

"But none of this applies to me: I am not vain, I have plenty of time here, and I am definitely not addicted to stress. I used to be a kind of workaholic but that passion has long evaporated. So what can I do about stress out here?"

"You said you worry about Nyala, about your future. Why? Are you imagining getting sick? O dying soon out here?"

I nodded.

"But none of these dark scenarios have occurred yet. You are healthy, feeling better with each passing day, Nyala is doing just fine. So all these stressors are just in your head, they are the products of your imagination, and most likely they will never occur."

"Yes, but—"

"Listen. Just do this. Whenever a dark thought intrudes into your mind, think of something positive you have recently experienced. I bet that the positive thoughts will easily overwhelm anything negative that might be bothering you."

I reflected on my earlier life back home. There it was only too easy to become enslaved by stress. In my ambitions I oftentimes made commitments that were unreasonable and could take more than one lifetime to accomplish. The common root of most of my stressors was time—or rather, the lack of it. Why was there such a chronic shortage of time? Time was a resource that could be turned into many things, including money. At the same time, technology was constantly bombarding me with new enticing products, which I felt I needed and richly deserved. Much of my time was also invested into personal achievements for the sake of illusory fame and power over others. And just as there is no limit to how much money one can make, there is also no limit on fame and power. All these pursuits contributed to my divorce, the fact that I had no children, no hobbies, no social life, and no one I could really call a close friend. I was trapped in a boundless web of over-commitment.

"I think I will be all right after all," I said after a long pause. "The few months out here have completely changed my priorities, which I assume was part of your plan for taking me away from my old life."

X smiled graciously.

"Here you easily liberated yourself from unreasonable expectations, something that would be extremely hard to do in your old life. You can see and accept that your present life can be improved but only by small steady increments. Only very few people become millionaires, Nobel Price recipients, or national leaders. This requires talent, luck, and hard work. Unfortunately, you can only influence the last of the three; talent and luck are largely beyond your control. This may not be fair, but fairness is an artificial concept foreign to nature. You simply have to learn to accept the fact that everyone is different and set your goals relative to your abilities and to the stage of life you are in. Accept that you do not need the biggest loan your bank will grant you, which you then immediately spend on the most expensive car or other luxury nonsense. The resulting excitement is very short-lived and only leads down a path of more loans, more struggles, and more stress."

As X spoke, I could see the fallacies of my earlier desires and aspirations unfold in a stream of delusions. How different from my highest goal at present—to bake better bread.

***

That night, I went to bed early. I felt unusually tired, my arms and legs seemed to be made out of lead pipes. I fell asleep instantly but woke up a few hours later, drenched in sweat. It was a cool night yet my skin was burning. I threw away my blanket and tried to get up; I desperately needed to drink something, but my muscles would not obey me. I looked around in the darkness. I could make out the black silhouettes of my table, the open window. I was not dreaming, I was sick.

"Nyala," I called out, but my voice was too thin. I tried again, putting all my strength behind it.

She stirred.

"Papa?" she asked sleepily. I taught her this word and she happily used it.

"Water," I said.

She did not respond. "Nyala, darling. I need a cup of water."

She got up and came over to my bed. I took her hand.

"You hot," she said.

"Please get me water, I am too weak to get up."

She walked over to the corner where we kept a jug of water and I heard her filling a cup. I rolled over to my side, propped my head up on my hand and tried to drink from the cup that Nyala held up to my lips. I spilled much of it but the cool liquid made me feel better.

I took Nyala's hand in mine. "I feel sick, my little darling. You must help me."

"What I do?" she asked.

"Get a piece of cloth, make it wet, and put it on my forehead."

She followed my instructions and I felt the coolness of the water drawing me back into sleep.

When I woke up, the sun was already shining through the window. Nyala was still kneeling next to my bed; I felt the wet rag on my forehead.

"You up," she said, touching my hand. "You better?"

I was still hot and lifting my arm to stroke Nyala's hair was a strenuous task.

She stood up and I heard her preparing something in the kitchen corner. She returned after a while with a bowl and a spoon.

"You eat," she said and touched my lips with the spoon. A few drops of a broth dribbled into my mouth.

"No." I shook my head. "I can't." I closed my eyes. Red and green dots were dancing wildly in front of me. I was in hell.

I must have slept a long time because when I opened my eyes, it was nighttime again. I felt Nyala's delicate body next to me. She was breathing peacefully. What woke me up was an almost unbearable headache. A meat grinder was working its way through my brain. Despite several blankets that Nyala must have piled up over me, I was still shivering uncontrollably. I reached out and pulled Nyala toward me. Her body felt like a block of ice against by burning skin.

As the night dragged on, fear began to spread though my body. Was I dying? I was supposed to die from cancer, not from some mysterious tropical disease. But how could I? What would become of Nyala?

People turned to God when facing hopeless desperation. Was there a God? If there was any higher being in this universe, controlling its motions, he couldn't allow such injustice. I had never prayed in my life. I never felt the need for it, always felt in control of my life. But my cancer diagnosis ripped my confidence to shreds and my stay in Africa made me feel less significant than a speck of dust in the universe.

"Dear God," I heard myself whisper. "If you can hear me, do not abandon Nyala. She needs me. Grant me more time to set her on her own path. I ask nothing for me. I have already had a good life and will gladly surrender it. But she is just a small helpless fragile child."

***

When I woke up again, it was daytime and Nyala wasn't next to me. I looked across the room. She was not in her bed either. In panic, I rose and called out for her. Seconds later the door flew open and she ran in.

"Papa," she cried with boundless joy, "you up."

She ran up to me and pressed herself against me so forcefully that I fell back on the bed and she on top of me. We remained lying there in a tight embrace, her soft cheek pressed against mine and her long black hair covering my face.

I ran a quick self-check. My headache was gone, I wasn't feeling particularly hot or cold, I was able to move my arms and legs without much difficulty.

"It was you," I said and stroked Nyala's supple back in gratitude. "You saved my life."

X visited me the following night.

"You got me worried," he said, shaking his head. "For some time I thought you wouldn't make it."

"So why didn't you save me?"

X laughed. "I am not God, you know."

"I know, but you seem to have powers beyond the normal."

"You are mistaken, my friend. I am nothing, just an illusion produced inside your head. Haven't you discovered that yet? No one saved you but you yourself."

I thought about this for a moment. "I prayed—is that what you mean?"

"In a way."

"But I don't even believe in God."

X smiled. "So why did you pray?"

"I was just desperate, and delirious. I don't believe in any personal deity that watches my every move, castigates me when I am bad, saves me when I pray. Why would the creator of the universe worry about trifling details of every human ant wandering about this planet?"

"And yet you prayed. Why?"

I sighed. Why did I? Something did change for me that night. I always believed that there was something much larger than the world we inhibit, a higher power that determined the course of the universe, someone who created the laws that allowed nature to function.

"My prayer was not a desperate call to a higher power to save me," I said after a while. "Yet I recognized that It existed, that there was something so great that we will never be able to grasp it with our limited reason, yet each of us is part of it, and it is part of each of us. My prayer was my admission of my ignorance, and my arrogance. I became humble and I accepted whatever might happen to me."

"You have acquired great wisdom through your ordeal," X said. "You prayed, but it was not the prayer that saved you. There was no one listening and judging you. Instead you reached a level of spirituality, which resides deep within you, and which no biological process will ever be able to explain. You have called upon powers beyond our visible and conscious world and have come another step closer to a healthy and fulfilling life."

I wanted to ask many more questions about this mysterious experience but when I looked up, X was already gone. The first birds had just begun to announce the arrival of a new day.

***

Today I had an experience that was almost magical. I went on my usual walk around the Bush but got further afield than usual. The vegetation became rather dense and lush, almost a rainforest. I spotted a bird that I had not seen before. It was perched on a branch high on a tree and I wouldn't have noticed it if it hadn't called out. It started to sing, but the sounds it was emitting were not too pleasing; it sounded more like urgent calls, as if trying to make me notice it. It was an inconspicuous little bird, the size of a starling, with a dull brown back and a cream-colored chest.

I resumed my walk but to my surprise, the bird showed up again in front of me. It landed on another high branch and while flapping his wings and hopping around, it kept emitting its strange squeaks. I watched it for a while and the bird seemed to be paying attention to me. Curious.

I continued along the path and the bird kept pace with me, flying ahead a few yards and waiting for me to catch up. I wasn't sure what to make of this. Then I vaguely remembered having read about birds that guide other animals, and even people, to find something. But what? Water? Fruit?

I decided to follow the bird's lead. It took off in a different direction than where I was headed, but it kept waiting for me every few moments to catch up. We must have walked for more than a mile and I began to worry about finding my way back. Suddenly the bird descended from the treetop and sat on a branch low to the ground. As I approached it, I perceived the buzzing of bees. Then I discovered the bird was guiding me toward honey.

The bees were flying in and out of a narrow crack in a large rock. I looked at the bird—it was still sitting on the same branch, observing me. I cautiously approach the entrance to the bees' nest. Some became agitated at my intrusion and I quickly retreated to avoid getting stung.

I looked at the bird. "Now what?"

There was no further help forthcoming; I would have to improvise. I gathered a few dry branches and leaves and lit a small fire. When it started to die down, I swept the hot embers onto a large leaf and covered them with wet moss. I placed the heavily smoking bundle on the ground just under the entrance to the bees' nest. The heavy white smoke penetrated the nest and the nervous buzzing calmed down. Cautiously, I approached the nest again. The bees were now slow and lethargic. I peeked inside the hole. Just inches from the entrance was a large honeycomb. I reached in and pulled it out. It was covered with bees but I managed to flick them off, suffering only a few stings. The effort was worth the trouble—the comb was dripping with delicious honey, which I began to suck out of the waxy enclosure.

I threw the leftovers on the ground and reached in to get two more combs. I carefully wrapped them into a large leaf to take them home for Nyala. What a delight it would be to spread this delicacy on a slice of her crusty bread.

In my excitement, I completely forgot about my guide-bird but his efforts were clearly not altruistic. As I started to leave, I saw him happily devouring the leftovers of the wax and honey that I left behind on the ground. I couldn't stop to marvel at this most curious symbiosis.

When I shared my excitement about this wonderful experience with X, he was not surprised.

"This is nothing rare in nature," he explained. "Many species, both animals and plants, depend on each other for survival. Many birds pick insects from the furs and skins of other animals. The birds get a tasty treat, the animals get rid of annoying parasites. There are birds who dare to venture even into the open mouths of crocodiles. In the long run, the crocodiles benefit from the dental cleaning more than from snapping their deadly jaws shut when a bird enters."

"Fascinating," I had to admit. "But how did animals learn to behave this way? How would a bird learn to lead a human to a bees' nest?"

"Nature is a very patient experimenter. Small coincidences can be reinforced and magnified when both parties benefit. How did dogs become our best friends? Some daring wolves started to hang around our campfires, they provided an early warning system against other predators and in exchange they got some scraps of our food. Both parties benefited and through many generations of adaptation they evolved into our present companions."

"I see. What other arrangements like that exist in nature?"

"There are too many to count. In the ocean, for example, the clownfish dwell among the tentacles of sea anemones. The clown fish protects the anemone from anemone-eating fish and in turn the stinging tentacles of the anemone protect the clownfish from its predators. Then think of insects. They pollinate most plants in exchange for tasty nectar. The earth would be in great trouble without insects. Another example are certain ants that nest inside the thorns of acacia trees. In exchange for shelter, the ants protect the acacias from attacks by herbivores. Speaking of herbivores, many species, like antelopes, sheep, or even cows, host bacteria in their stomachs that help them digest cellulose, which enables them to live off grasses. Do I need to go on?"

"No need, but this idea of hosting bacteria inside an organism is strange. I have always thought of bacteria as something linked with a disease, something to be avoided."

"And that is very naïve thinking, my friend," X continued. "There are trillions of bacteria living on your body and especially inside it all the time. Some can be harmful, but in a healthy body they are vastly outnumbered by bacteria that are benign or even essential for good health. Your digestive tract, from your lips all the way to the opposite end, is teeming with bacteria that help you digest, that produce certain vitamins, or that regulate your immune system and actually protect you from disease-causing bacteria."

"I have never thought of bacteria in a positive sense."

"Of course not," X continued. "You have been taught to eliminate them whenever and wherever possible. The obsessive hygiene of your civilized world that likes to bath everything in anti-bacterial chemicals carries much of the blame for the many chronic maladies. But an even greater sin committed against your beneficial bacteria is neglect."

"Neglect?" I marveled in disbelief. "Not only am I prohibited from exterminating bacteria but I am supposed to nurture and care for them? How would I do that?"

"Bacteria are living organisms, they need to eat. And they can only eat what you give them, that is, what you eat yourself. Most beneficial bacteria need large amounts and a great variety of fibers. If you live on burgers, french fries, and milkshakes, they starve, and their place is taken up by those that enjoy your junk food and that will cause you harm."

This was most revealing. My diet had changed radically from what I used to eat back home. I felt great and was experiencing none of the digestive annoyances I used to combat with antacids and other medications.

X could read my thoughts.

"In your new environment," he concluded, "you were able to restore the natural balance of bacteria not only on your skin but must importantly within your gut. Your microbiome has once again become a healthy ecosystem and is repaying you generously with protection and a deep sense of well-being."

***

It had been eleven months and twenty three days since I came to my new home. I became very familiar with my surroundings; I knew every bush and every creek as if I had grown up with them. I knew the daily routine of the birds and lizards, and the nightly buzzing and chirping of all insects.

I decided it was time to venture even further afield to find out what lay beyond the horizon of my one-day walks. I packed a small bag with dried fruits and some bread left over from last night and I explained to Nyala what I was about to do. Her high forehead crumpled into furrows of worries but she said nothing, just eyed me cautiously as I made my preparations.

The land to the west was flat as far as I could see and so I decided to head east, toward a range of bluish mountains far on the horizon. It was still early morning, the sun had barely made it appearance, as I began my walk toward my chosen destination. According to my calendar, it was now mid-March, close to the equinox, and so I knew the sun would travel in a straight line from east to west, passing directly overhead. That was important because it would allow me to find my way back should I have gotten lost.

I walked quietly for several hours, still paying attention to my surroundings, but my mind kept wandering in many directions, trying to anticipate what I might discover tomorrow. When the sun passed its zenith and began its slow descent toward the west, I reached the boundary of my known territory. In front of me lay terra incognita—areas into which I couldn't venture in a single day without running the risk of having to spend the night in the open.

There was no major change in the landscape at first but as the blueness of the mountains came closer and became more pronounced, I began to notice a gradual undulation of the surrounding savannah. Later I entered a large plateau studded with graceful junipers and carved by dry riverbeds into a rugged landscape of steep hills and deep depressions filled with impenetrable vegetation.

It was almost evening when I began to think about a suitable place to spend the night. I climbed a small ridge to see further ahead and, as I was reaching the summit, I perceived a feigned unexpected noise that sounded like human laughter. I stopped and closed my eyes to better focus my hearing. I heard nothing more than the familiar sounds of nature. I resumed my ascent—and there it was again: a sound reminiscent of female laughter far in the distance. It couldn't be. I felt my heart beating, not from fear but from excitement. I had not heard a human voice other than Nyala's in many months and it felt surprisingly alien and nostalgic at the same time.

With great caution I negotiated the final stretch to the top of the ridge and peaked passed the previously hidden line of sight. The land continued in an endless series of gentle ridges and shallow valleys all the way to the horizon. And there it was again, undeniable this time: the playful banter of female voices somewhere not too far from me. I listened in hypnotic captivation. There were at least four or five different voices. I also heard something like water rushing bye. For a moment I thought I was hallucinating—the result of my exile from civilization and too much sun exposure during my long march. But it was real, and it was very close.

I decided to investigate. With extreme caution, I descended into the shallow valley in front of me. I tried to keep hidden behind the countless bushes but could see no one keeping a watch. As soon as I reached the top of the next low hill, a scene of idyllic beauty opened up in front of me. A lively stream ran down the length of the valley floor, forcing its way in between huge boulders and skipping over a myriad of rocks in a symphony of gurgling sounds. Through the curtain of trees lining the banks I spotted several women playing in the water, laughing playfully as they splashed each other. They were dressed in colorful t-shirts and shorts that clung to their glistening bodies like outlandish wetsuits.

I watched for a long time, unable to decide what to do. The unexpected sight of a bearded stranger would probably frighten them. Perhaps I should have just retreated quietly and avoid any danger. I wondered where all the men might be. But my legs were frozen. They refused to take me away. The unexpected sight of young women after months of solitude was gripping my brain like an iron claw from a sci-fi movie. I was mesmerized and I was paralyzed.

When the sun began to lose its strength, the women stepped out on the river bank, pressed out the water from their skirts and hair, and while continuing their unintelligible banter, started to walk in the direction of where I lay hidden. I panicked. Without standing up, I tried to slither backwards, away from the direction of their path. The group veered off as they approached my hiding place but they were so close that I could hear the leaves rustle under their feet. I kept my body pressed down to the ground, watching only their bare feet through the openings in the foliage. Slowly their voices trailed off and I dared to raise myself onto my knees, but I misjudged the distance. As I raised my head, I found myself staring into the eyes of a woman whose face suddenly appeared just a few feet in front of me. She froze, only her hand flew up to cover her mouth, stifling a scream. For a few seconds she kept staring at me through the eyes of a startled gazelle. I slowly raised my hand in an awkward signal of peace. She let her hand drop, revealing a mouth still half-open. Then her head turned and she was gone.

I raised myself into a standing position and kept listening to the sounds of the surrounding forest. There were only the customary squeaks and chirps of the insects. When I was sure that the women were not coming back, I walked to the water's edge, took off my clothes and immersed myself in the stream to wash off the dust and the fatigue of the long day, but the vision of the bathing women kept swirling in my head as a swarm of restless bees.

X walked out of the forest just when I was getting ready to

go to sleep.

"X," I called out. "Where have you been for so long?"

X smiled as he settled down on the patch of grass next to me.

"You didn't need me and I hate to intrude."

"So why today?"

"I see that you need some council. You seem restless and confused. Tell me what you are feeling now."

I thought for a while. What was I feeling?

"I am greatly enjoying my new life," I said slowly. "Especially now that Nyala is with me ..."

"But?"

I didn't answer, so X picked up the trail of my thoughts.

"You feel lonely. Something important is missing. There is a hole in your life and you just came to realize it this afternoon."

I nodded. "I grew up in the city, always surrounded by people. I am not fit to lead the life of a hermit."

"No one is. We are social animals, and we need the presence of other humans to be sane. We need their voices, their touch, even their annoyances to feel alive."

I woke up but thought I was still dreaming. X was gone and in his place was a woman, watching me sleep. The sun was behind her back, creating a surreal halo around her black hair. I had to shield my eyes to look at her. It was the same face I saw yesterday in the forest. When she saw that I was awake, she smiled.

"Good morning," she said in a serene voice.

I looked around. We were alone. And no, I was no longer dreaming.

"Who are you?" I asked apprehensively.

"I am Kaila." Her teeth formed two perfect arches of pearls as she spoke.

"I'm Richard," I said and rose onto my elbow to better see her. She was sitting in a lotus position: her back straight, and her hands resting in her lap. She wore a bright yellow dress with large red and green flowers.

"I'm sorry about yesterday," I continued. "I didn't mean to frighten you. I just didn't know what to do."

"It's ok," she said calmly. "I already told my people about it. They know about you."

"Who knows?"

"Our elders. They knew that you live in the Karango Valley. And they think you are a good man," she said. "Not dangerous."

I asked her why they never came to see me but she didn't know. The elders had never mentioned me to the young people, perhaps to protect me from curious visitors. But I was not alone after all. Someone had been aware of my existence all this time.

We talked for a while.

"It must be a lonely life you are leading," she said.

"It is, but I'm not complaining. It is a small price to pay for being alive. But I am not alone."

"Oh? Who is there with you?"

"Do you know X?" I asked.

She shook her head. "I have never heard that name mentioned before."

"What about Nyala?"

Perhaps she was lost from their village, or somewhere nearby, I thought.

Again she shook her head. "Who is she?"

"A small girl I am taking care of."

She raised her eyebrows, demanding more information. I told her all I knew about Nyala and her late grandmother.

"That is so sad," she said. "You must be a good man."

"I was very fortunate that she came into my life. It gives me a purpose." Then, without thinking about possible consequences I blurted out. "You should meet her. Can you come with me to my home sometime?"

She lowered her eyes and remained silent for a long time before speaking again. "I would like that. But… I need to ask my family."

"Of course. That's not a problem for me. Just go back now. I can wait."

She leaned forward and touched my hand. Her palm felt soft and warm. "I will be back with my answer tomorrow morning. Can you wait that long?"

"What is one day in a lifetime? I will be happy to wait for you."

"I'll bring you food tomorrow again." With that, she rose and disappeared in the dense foliage.

It was already getting dark, so I ate the rest of the food Kaila had brought me and found a suitable place to spend the night. Sleep didn't come easily that night as I kept reliving the dialog with Kaila in my mind and thinking what tomorrow might bring.

Kaila returned shortly after sunrise and she woke me by gently squeezing my hand. She was all smiles.

Before I could wish her a good morning, she already confirmed that she wanted to come with me today.

"I am so happy to hear that," I said. "All night I was hoping you would say that."

"I have to see the little girl," she said. "What was her name again?"

"Nyala," I said. "That's what she told me when we first met."

"I need to speak with her, to find out why and how she ended up in your place."

I gathered my belongings and we set off on the long march back to my hut. We spoke on and off to satisfy our mutual curiosities. I explained how I ended up in this part of the world and what my daily life was like. She told me about the daily life in her village and her aspirations.

"My greatest wish is to live a healthy and peaceful life," she said. "Nothing more but also nothing less. I hope to find a good husband and have children. Not too many," she smiled bashfully, "but enough to keep me busy for the rest of my life."

"Is that really all you wish for?" I probed. "You don't care about money, being able to buy nice things, conveniences in the home, a car maybe? Or to travel to other places?"

She shook her head. "Too many things make you a slave. When you want something beyond your means, you work harder, you become angry and frustrated, you try to save and cause your health and your family to suffer for months or years. Then when you get what you wanted, you are excited for a while, but very soon you are back where you started and already thinking about the next thing you need to be happy."

I was impressed by her intuitive understanding of what ancient philosophies, like Buddhism, were trying to teach us.

"So you don't care at all about any material possessions?" I asked.

"Don't be silly. Of course I care about money," she continued, "but you only need enough to have a comfortable place to live and healthy food to eat. Anything beyond that is a waste that will not make you happy."

It was already late afternoon when we reached the vicinity of my hut. This area I knew only too well and I told Kaila that we would be arriving soon. When we ascended the last hill, I could make out the dark silhouette of my hut against the setting sun. I shielded my eyes against the glare to see if I could spot Nyala. She was not outside so we resumed our walk, spurred by the excitement of the expected encounter.

Once we were in shouting distance, I called Nyala's name. She appeared in the doorway and as soon as she recognized me, she started to run toward us. A few minutes later she stood in front of us, panting, and observing Kaila with great curiosity.

"Nyala?" Kaila asked before I could attempt an introduction.

"Awo," Nyala replied shyly.

"Yigebahali?" Kaila continued.

At this, Nyala's face lit up and she burst forth with a long narrative of which I didn't understand a single word. They kept talking for a while and I could only guess from their emotions and gestures that Nyala was explaining to Kaila the curious circumstances of her arrival here.

I was burning with curiosity to find out Nyala's story but it was getting late and Kaila promised to tell me everything in the morning.

I could not fall asleep that night for many hours, thinking about the events of the past two days and feeling very unsure of what should happen next. When my mind finally let go of the revolving thoughts, I fell into a deep sleep and woke up only when the sun made the air in the hut uncomfortably hot. I was alone. The women must have gotten up early, I concluded, and went out. I ate a quick breakfast and stepped out to see how they were getting along. They were nowhere to be seen so I called for them, first Nyala, then Kaila, but there was no reply. I listened carefully and tried again, lauder. Still no reply.

I walked down toward the brook, the most likely place where Nyala would have taken Kaila. I called out again a few times but still no reply. At this point I became concerned. Why would they venture so far from the house at this early hour and without letting me know?

I made a larger circle around the house, checking all places we normally visited with Nyala but they seemed to have vanished without a trace.

There was nothing else I could do, so I returned to the hut and waited. Could they have been lost? I dismissed that possibility since Nyala knew every shrub and every anthill in our vicinity. Could they have been attacked by a lion? This again was a very unlikely scenario, given the time of day and the fact that the last lioness I had encountered was the one on my first day's trek.

I made another round in the afternoon, venturing as far as I could imagine anyone going, but without success.

That night was one of the most distressing since my arrival here. The uncertainly of what might have happened was grinding on my conscience like a slowly revolving millstone.

My desperation was compounded by the fact that just yesterday I had made the last mark of the twelfth row on my wall calendar. I was planning to celebrate one year of my survival in my new home. Three hundred and sixty-five days of peace and tranquility, and almost as many days of happiness with Nyala. She was the only person I really cared about. She was my family, and now she was gone.

I desperately needed someone to consult with. Fortunately X appeared exactly when I was succumbing to my deepest anxiety and helplessness. He knew what I wanted to ask him and stopped me before I could unleash my barrage of questions at him

"I have good news for you," he said.

"Where are they?" I blurted out. "What has happened?"

"I am not talking about Nyala or Kaila. There is something more important to talk about."

"No," I objected, "there is absolutely nothing more important right now."

"Ok, but tell me something first. How did you envision your future? Stay here forever? Alone with Nyala? Would that be a good life for her?"

I had frequently contemplated those questions. Despite our comfortable life here, thoughts of our future started to intrude with increasing urgency. There was not much I missed from my previous life. I could easily imagine remaining here indefinitely. But it didn't seem right for Nyala. She was growing up and she needed other people, children and adults, not just an aging father.

"When I met Kaila," I said tentatively, "the thought of letting her take Nyala to her people did cross my mind."

"That thought is a testament to your generosity, selflessness, and wisdom," X said.

"But where are they?"

"Your thought has already been turned into reality," X said slowly.

"What? They have left? Without even saying goodbye?" I could not believe that this was the end of my experience of being a father.

"It's better that way," X said. "No tears, no promises of staying in touch, no heartbreak for either of you."

I sighed deeply. So that was it. This experience was ending just as abruptly as it began. I felt my life slowly reconnecting with the first days of my arrival. The circle seemed to be closing.

"What's the good news you spoke about," I reminded X after a long pause.

"I think you are beginning to guess it," X resumed. "You have been here for exactly one year now."

I nodded, still unsure where he was headed with this preamble.

"You are not only alive but seemingly very healthy," he said. "Why?"

I asked myself that question a million times. What did it? Why were the oncologists wrong in their prediction?

I shrugged. "I think I have been too busy to die."

"You give a flippant answer yet deep down you know that you are right. Let me tell you something about modern medicine and why it is so limited. Just a few thousand years ago, humans were humble, insignificant creatures, barely surviving on this earth. With time you became arrogant and you thought you could dominate nature. You believe in science, you laugh at earlier generations' attempts to cure diseases, yet you fail to see how little you understand yourselves. You believe in your chemistry as much as earlier healers believed in leeches and bloodletting, and you fail to recognize that future generations will be laughing at you."

He paused to let his words sink in.

"I accept that," I said, "but can you explain how that saved me?"

"Yes and no. The yes-part is this: you returned to an environment and a lifestyle for which your body was designed by millions of years of evolution. You have not changed much in the last few thousand years; you are still the hunter and gatherer, and the early farmer. Sitting in an office chair all day long, eating processed foods, worrying about deadlines, and being totally disconnected from raw nature and even from your fellow homo sapiens is something very unnatural. It made you sick. By coming here, you gave your body a chance to fight back."

"And the no-part?" I asked.

"I cannot tell you how your body did it. It just did. We must accept that there are powers that we will never understand, much less control. That's faith."

"And your role in all of this," I asked.

"Have you not figured it out yet," X said. "I am your inner guide, your subconscious mind, I am nature itself. You have always turned to me for advice and I have always given you what's best for you."

We both fell silent. Then I again remembered his opening line.

"You still haven't told me what the good news is."

"You can go home now."

"But why should I go back now that Nyala is gone?" I asked. "This is my true home. It is the best home I have ever had."

"True, but you still have to go back," he said with finality.

"Tell me why. You just told me that civilization had almost killed me. So?"

"First, you are now strong enough to go back. Your experiences here have reprogrammed your mind sufficiently to withstand the illusory and dangerous temptation of civilization and to lead a healthy and natural life even within the environment you came from a year ago."

"And second?" I asked, anxious about what else I may have to face.

"There is something important you need to do," X said. "A final step to complete your cure."

I was not happy with this ominous pronouncement but said nothing.

"Do you still remember how you ended up here?" he asked.

"Of course, the initial anonymous phone call I almost rejected," I recalled.

"Exactly. But you cannot be the last person to benefit from the cure. You need to pass it on to continue the chain."

I began to grasp what he meant but let him continue.

"You need to find two people who are terminally ill, just like you were, and convince them to come here."

"Why two?"

"If every saved person recruits two more at the end of the year, then there will be over one thousand people saved in only ten years, and over a million in twenty. Do the calculation if you don't believe me."

"I understand," I said with finality. "The price for my life is to save the life of others. I accept."

ABOUT THE AUTHORS

Lubomir Bic, PhD, is a professor of Computer Science in the Donald Bren School of Information and Computer Sciences at the University of California, Irvine.

Zuzana Bic DrPH, MUDr.(MD), is a Senior Lecturer and the Director of Student Experience in Public Health Practice in the Department of Population Health and Disease Prevention, Susan and Henry Samueli College of Health Sciences, University of California, Irvine